Low-Calorie Foods and Food Ingredients

Low-Calorie Foods and Food Ingredients

Edited by

RIAZ KHAN
Scientific Director
POLY-biòs LBT
Trieste

BLACKIE ACADEMIC & PROFESSIONAL
An Imprint of Chapman & Hall

London · Glasgow · New York · Tokyo · Melbourne · Madras

Published by Blackie Academic & Professional, an imprint of Chapman & Hall, Wester Cleddens Road, Bishopbriggs, Glasgow G64 2NZ

Chapman & Hall, 2–6 Boundary Row, London SE1 8HN, UK

Blackie Academic & Professional, Wester Cleddens Road, Bishopbriggs, Glasgow G64 2NZ, UK

Chapman & Hall Inc., 29 West 35th Street, New York NY10001, USA

Chapman & Hall Japan, Thomson Publishing Japan, Hirakawacho Nemoto Building, 6F, 1–7–11 Hirakawa-cho, Chiyoda-ku, Tokyo 102, Japan

DA Book (Aust.) Pty Ltd, 648 Whitehorse Road, Mitcham 3132, Victoria, Austalia

Chapman & Hall India, R. Seshadri, 32 Second Main Road, CIT East, Madras 600 035, India

First edition 1993

© 1993 Chapman & Hall

Typeset in 10/12pt Times, by Falcon Graphic Art, Surrey
Printed in Great Britain by St Edmundsbury Press, Bury St. Edmunds, Suffolk

ISBN 0 7514 0004 1

A catalogue record for this book is available from the British Library

Library of Congress Cataloging-in-Publication data

Low-Calorie foods and food ingredients / edited by Riaz Khan.--1st ed.
    p.   cm.
  Includes bibliographical references and index.
  ISBN 0–7514–0004–1
  1. Low-fat foods. 2. Low-calorie diet.   I. Khan, Riaz, 1939–   .
TP451.L67L69   1993
664'.63--dc20   93-3183
                                                                     CIP

Contributors

Dr G. Annison

CSIRO Division of Human Nutrition, Glenthorne Laboratory, Majors Road, O'Halloran Hill, SA 5158, Australia

Dr R.N. Antenucci

Formerly Product Development, McNeil Specialty Products. Now at AVEBE America, Inc., 4 Independence Way, CN5307, Princeton, NJ 08543–5370, USA

Dr R.L. Barndt

Product Development, McNeil Specialty Products, 501 George Street, PO Box 2400, New Brunswick, NJ 08903-2400, USA

Dr C. Bertocchi

POLY-biòs LBT, Area di Ricerca, Padriciano 99, 1-34012 Trieste, Italy

Professor J.E. Blundell

Department of Psychology, University of Leeds, Leeds LS2 9JT, UK

Dr F.R.J. Bornet

Nutrition and Health Department, Eridania Béghin-Say, Gruppo Ferruzzi, 54 Avenue Hoche 75008, Paris, France

Mrs C. Bressan

Laboratoire de Chimie Physique Industrielle, Faculté des Sciences, Université de Reims Champagne-Ardenne, BP347, 51062 Reims Cedex, France

Dr C. de Graaf

Department of Human Nutrition, University of Wageningen, PO Box 8129, 6700EV Wageningen, The Netherlands

Professor L. Hough

20 Newstead Way, Wimbledon, London, SW19 5HR, UK

Dr R. Khan

POLY-biòs LBT, Area di Ricerca, Padriciano 99, 1-34012 Trieste, Italy

Dr M.G.Lindley

Lintech, Reading University Innovation Centre, Philip Lyle Building, PO Box 68, Whiteknights, Reading, RG6 2BX, UK

Professor M. Mathlouthi

Laboratoire de Chimie Physique Industrielle, Faculté des Sciences, Université de Reims Champagne-Ardenne, BP347, 51062 Reims Cedex, France

Dr S.V. Molinary Tate & Lyle Speciality Sweeteners, PO Box 68, Whiteknights, Reading RG6 2BX, UK

Mr G. Urquhart Tate & Lyle Speciality Sweeteners, PO Box 68, Whiteknights, Reading PG6 2BX, UK

Contents

5 Fat replacer ingredients and the markets for fat-reduced foods   77
M.G.LINDLEY

6 Fat and calorie-modified bakery products   106
R.L. BARNDT and R.N. ANTENUCCI

Editorial introduction

R. KHAN

It is now generally recognised that a high-calorie diet with inadequate physical activity results in overweight or obesity, which in turn could lead to diseases like non-insulin dependent diabetes, hypertension, atherosclerotic cardiovascular disease, endometriol cancer and gall-stones. Obesity, the storage of excessive amounts of fat, has become a major health problem. In the USA more than 30% of the population over 25 years of age is overweight and on a European scale it is estimated that approximately 40 million people are obese or over-weight. Body fatness can roughly be measured in terms of 'body mass index' (BMI), that is weight (kg) divided by height (m). A BMI value between 20 and 25 is considered to be average and above 30 is classed as overweight or obese.

In order to maintain an average weight it is essential to strike a right energy balance, that is the energy input is equal to the energy output. In the case of overweight or obese individuals a negative energy balance has to be achieved by low-energy intake, without reducing the essential nutrients such as minerals, trace elements and vitamins, and by increased energy expenditure. The Western diet and comfortable lifestyle result in excessive amounts of energy, contributing to weight gain and ill health. With this concern in mind, health authorities in most of the advanced countries have proposed dietary guidelines, for example in the UK the Department of Health has produced an excellent report entitled *Dietary Reference Values for Food Energy and Nutrients for the United Kingdom.*

The apparent connection between diet and health has increased the awareness for 'healthier' eating. The diet with 'reduced fat', 'reduced cholesterol' and 'enhanced fibre' is in vogue. This trend is reflected in the increased markets for low-fat dairy products and 'lite' or 'light' soft drinks, in particular in the USA and in Europe. There is little doubt that the consumer preference is still for foods and drinks with quality texture, flavour and taste. Most of the market surveys carried out in recent years indicate that the demand for 'healthier' food will increase but not at the cost of quality and taste. This presents the industry with a challenge and an opportunity to develop new technologies to produce consumer acceptable low-calorie food products. It also offers the opportunity to search for new and novel additives and food ingredients. A decision to develop a new food additive will have to take into account the high cost involved in toxicological trials, long lead-time required for the safety approval, process development and market research. As a rough estimate, the time required for a product like a high-intensity sweetener from the initial discovery to its introduction to the market is about fifteen years and the cost could be between 15 and 20 million pounds sterling. However, judging from the ever increasing sales of low-calorie products with high-intensity sweeteners, fat substitutes and bulking materials, such an investment in research and development will be justifiable.

Low-calorie foods can be divided into ingredients such as carbohydrates, proteins and fat, and additives such as high-intensity sweeteners, fat substitutes and bulking materials like polydextrose. When a new food additive or ingredient is developed it is the responsibility of the company to obtain the seal of approval of safety in use from the regulatory authority of the country where the product is to be marketed. The main regulatory authorities in the advanced countries are: the Food and Drug Administration (FDA) of the USA, the Food Advisory Committee (FAC) of the UK, the FAO/WHO Joint Expert Committee on Food Additives (JECFA), the EC Scientific Committee for Food (SCF), the Health Protection Branch (HPB) of Canada, the Life Hygiene Bureau, Ministry of Health and Welfare (Japan), the National Food Authority (NFA) of Australia, the Food Standards Committee of New Zealand, the Codex Alimentarius Commission (CAC) and the Organisation of Economic Cooperation and Development (OECD).

Regulatory procedures for obtaining approval for additives that are to be used in small quantities, such as a high-intensity sweeteners, are adequately defined. In most of the European countries, the company which owns the product has first to prove the case for 'need' and then the case for 'safety-in-use'. In the USA it is not necessary to demonstrate the case for 'need'. The FDA 'Red Book' (*Toxicological Principles for the Safety Assessment of Direct Food Additives*), currently being revised, gives a comprehensive list of the type of studies required for submission for safety approval. Typically these include: (a) additive identification and characterisation; (b) use and the projected level of intake; and (c) toxicological data. The safety testings are carried out to a standard set by the FDA called Good Laboratory Practice (GLP). The tests include: acute toxicity (mouse, rat); genetic toxicology; metabolism and pharmacokinetics (rat, dog, man); sub-acute toxicity (rat, dog); reproductive toxicology, teratology (rat, rabbit); chronic toxicity, carcinogenicity (rat); biochemistry, immunology, studies on the impurities if required; ecotoxicology, biodegradability, environmental impact.

The responsibility for safety assessment and risk management of the product continues to lie with the regulatory authorities of the country where the approval has been granted. The risk evaluation of a food additive is based on the concept that any food given in large enough amounts can produce a deleterious effect on animals. In an attempt to quantify this potential for toxicity and to give sufficient margin for safety, JECFA has introduced an acceptable daily intake (ADI) level for food additives. For example, the ADI values granted for saccharin, aspartame, cyclamate, acesulfame-K and sucralose are 2.5, 40, 11, 9 and 3.5 mg kg^{-1} body weight per day, respectively. Chapter 2 on regulatory aspects of low-calorie food elaborates these points.

The additives that are to be consumed in large amounts, such as a fat replacement product like 'Olestra' or a new bulking material like 'polydextrose', present a more complex problem as far as the evaluation of their toxicity is concerned. Normal safety testing of an additive, such as a high-intensity sweetener, requires that the test animals are fed with a sufficiently high dosage in order to produce an effect and then on that basis an ADI value is calculated. In cases like 'Olestra' and 'polydextrose', which are not normally present in diet or metabolised to dietary constituents, such an approach will obviously not be applicable, or of any use, in calculating an ADI value. Due to these factors the regulatory authorities have not yet been able to produce any guidelines for toxicity trials for additives that are to be taken in food in large quantities. In the USA low-calorie food ingredients which are normally present in the diet or metabolised to dietary constituents are in general given the 'generally recognised as safe' (GRAS) status.

The consumers' preference for a low-calorie product is not only for a dietary purpose but also to allow choice of a low-calorie version of a normal food. In response to consumer demand, the industry has developed considerable knowledge and expertise in producing and using new low-calorie food ingredients and additives. The three main groups of commercially important low-calorie food ingredients and additives are: high-intensity sweeteners, low-calorie fats and bulking materials. The need for a book that will provide a comprehensive and up-to-date scientific and technological coverage of the subject is recognised here. In order to achieve this objective, world experts have combined their efforts to deal with most aspects of low-calorie products. The subjects to be discussed are: physiology and psychology, safety and toxicity, nutrition, process technology, physicochemical and functional properties, product formulations, and markets and market potential. The role of high-intensity sweeteners, carbohydrates and fats in the biological and behavioural responses involved in energy balance is discussed in chapter 1.

Sugar polyols, fructo-oligosaccharides and non-starch polysaccharides are 'natural' low-calorie bulking ingredients. Their role in low-calorie foods as bland carriers for flavour and to provide such essential properties as viscosity, texture or mouthfeel, clarity, and stability is well recognised. Chapters 3 and 4 deal with the chemistry, biochemistry and nutritional aspects of low-calorie bulk sweeteners and bulking ingredients.

Fats and oils are important ingredients of food, and they are also the main actors in the 'calorie game'. Fats provide roughly 9 kcal g^{-1} of energy, over twice that of protein or carbohydrates, fuelling the interest in developing fat replacement products with lower energy while retaining the functional and organoleptic properties of normal fats. Chapter 5 on low-calorie fats presents a panoramic view of the subject and critically evaluates the properties and market potential of non-metabolisable fat substitutes, such as 'Olestra' and 'polysiloxane', metabolisable low-calorie fats such as 'caprenin', which is expected to obtain GRAS status in the near future, carbohydrate-based fat replacements, such as modified starches and gums, and protein as fat replacers, such as 'Simplesse' and 'Lita'.

Consumer demand for low-calorie bakery products has led to many innovations and technological developments in this sector of the market. Recent market surveys carried out in the USA and the UK on low calorie-modified bakery products have been reviewed. Chapter 6 unravels the story of how the baking industry responded to consumer demand for low-calorie baked products. It deals with the products and product formulations, marketing, and forecasts the market potential for the use of new low-calorie ingredients and additives to develop high-quality low-calorie baked goods.

The commercial success story of Nutrasweet's low-calorie sweetener aspartame has spurred research and development on new high-intensity sweeteners throughout the world. The recent safety approvals of Hoechst's sweetener acesulfame-K by the FDA and Tate and Lyle's sweetener 'sucralose' in Canada has encouraged others who are working in the same field. Companies like Pfizer, Procter and Gamble, General Foods Corporation, Mitsui Toatsu Chemical Incorporation and Coca Cola are actively or defensively involved in this area, because it is believed that the market is large enough to allow many competitors to take part in the game. Chapter 7 on high-intensity sweeteners covers the structure, synthesis, sweetness quality, and toxicological status of all the approved sweeteners. Chapter 8 on low-calorie soft drinks describes the technical requirements for formulation of a soft drink where sucrose is replaced by artificial sweeteners. Other important issues dealt with are the marketing aspects, taste synergy between artificial sweeteners and sugars, the role of water packing, and the solution properties of soft drinks.

It is hoped that this book covering current research as well as future needs and prospects will help in furthering our understanding of low-calorie foods. This project would not have been possible without the commitment and the cooperation of the contributors which is gratefully acknowledged. My special thanks go to Karin, my wife, for checking the manuscripts with me and for her patience and encouragement. I wish to thank POLY-biòs LBT for providing the facilities, with particular thanks to Magdalena Gemperle for her secretarial assistance during the course of this work.

R.K.

1 Low-calorie foods: relevance for body weight control

J.E. BLUNDELL and C. de GRAAF

1.1 Overconsumption and low-calorie foods

Obesity now represents one of the major health problems in affluent technologically developed societies. The condition is prevalent and leads to an increased risk of a number of disorders (Garrow, 1992). Moreover, it appears that in some countries the frequency of obesity has increased during the 1980s. Therefore dieting, treatments and preventive measures appear to be having little or no impact on the control of body weight. Considering the processes underlying energy regulation in the obese, it has been suggested that the condition represents a disorder of appetite control rather than of energy expenditure (Prentice *et al.*, 1989). It is within this context that the actions of low-calorie foods should be evaluated.

The ways in which foods may increase the willingness to eat or satisfy our desire for further foods is an issue of great theoretical importance and of considerable practical significance in this last decade of the 20th century. Products whose palatability has been raised in order to promote consumption may have the potential for causing overnutrition. In addition new types of foods and additives are constantly being added to the food supply although often little is known about their effects on appetite. Consequently there is a considerable need to provide information about the appetite enhancing and satiating capacity of food items. First, knowledge of how the composition of food alters energy intake and food selection throws light upon the mechanisms of appetite control. Food itself can be used as an experimental tool to investigate the mode of operation of appetite mechanisms. Second, this knowledge can be used to develop a coherent strategy of nutritional intake for everyday use in the home, at work and in the clinic. Knowledge about the effects on appetite control exerted by particular components of food can help industry to provide appropriate foods for specific requirements and can allow the consumer rationally to select a suitable diet. Despite the importance of these issues, only a little is known about the satiating properties (or appetite enhancing capacity) of foods in general and only a few studies have examined the effects of individual food components.

Why have the above issues become particularly important in the last quarter of the 20th century? There are two prominent reasons. First, advances in food technology have made it possible to develop and produce foods with precisely defined sensory characteristics. These characteristics are designed to make foods particularly attractive to the consumer (the eater and the purchaser). At the same time it is clear that the sensory characteristics of foods can be manipulated quite independently of the nutrient or calorific content of food. This disengagement (or uncoupling) of the sensory and nutritional components of food is likely to have effects upon the control of appetite and the pattern of ingestion.

Second, in well developed economic cultures such as North America and Europe, the last ten years have seen increased attention directed to the problem of obesity and to the effects of excess weight on health. This concern has been reflected in the extent to which the media have promoted the doctrine of slimness, particularly amongst women. In turn these circumstances have provided the conditions for an epidemic of eating disorders ranging from mild but uncontrolled dieting to the disabling disorder of bulimia nervosa. A sizeable proportion of the population is, therefore, greatly concerned with body shape and weight and is actively attempting to undereat. This type of behaviour and the associated eating patterns brings to prominence the way in which foods satisfy hunger and provide for bodily requirements.

1.2   Appetite and the regulation of body weight

Appetite can be considered a phenomenon that links biological happenings (under the skin) with environmental events (beyond the skin). Indeed, the expression of appetite can be viewed as the end product of an intimate interaction between physiology and the environment (Blundell and Hill, 1986). Figure 1.1 illustrates how appetite is shaped by the principles of biological regulation and environmental adaptation. All living organisms require food (a nutrition supply) for growth and maintenance of tissues. This supply is achieved through behaviour commonly called eating. The expression of this behaviour is controlled according to the state of the biological system. A complex system of signals operates to ensure the appropriate direction and quality of this (eating) behaviour. The extension of Claude Bernard's principle of homeostasis to include behaviour is often referred to as the behavioural regulation of internal states (Richter, 1943). However, the expression of behaviour is also subject to environmental demands, and behaviour is therefore adapted in the face of particular circumstances.

In the case of human appetite, consideration should be given to the conscious and deliberate (external) control over behaviour. Human beings can decide to alter their own behaviour (eating) in order to meet particular objectives, for example, a display of moral conviction (political hunger strike) or a demonstration of aesthetic achievement (dieting). In both of

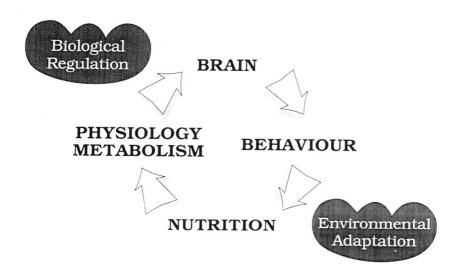

Figure 1.1 Scheme illustrating the place of eating behaviour in biological regulation and environmental adaptation.

these examples, eating is curtailed with an ensuing interruption of the nutritional supply. Regulatory mechanisms will tend to oppose this under-supply and generate a drive to eat. In the technically advanced cultures of Europe and the United States, the nutritional supply may be adjusted by the environment in another way. The existence of an abundant supply of palatable, high-energy dense food promotes overconsumption. This in turn, in an interaction with genetic susceptibility, leads to an increase in fat deposition (Bouchard, 1985). However, an oversupply of calories leading to deposition of fat does not generate a biological drive to undereat. Hence, the operation of the regulatory system is not symmetrical: there is a strong defence against undernutrition and only weak response to the effects of overnutrition.

1.3   Appetite control and the satiety cascade

The biological drive to eat can be linked with the satiating power of food. Satiating power, or satiating efficiency, is the term applied to the capacity of any consumed food to suppress hunger and to inhibit the onset of a further period of eating (Kissileff, 1984; Blundell *et al.*, 1987). Food brings about this effect by certain mediating processes that can be roughly classified as sensory, cognitive, post-ingestive, and post-absorptive. The operation of these processes is generated by the impact of food on physiological and biochemical mechanisms. Collectively these processes have been referred to as the satiety cascade (Blundell *et al.* 1988). The way that food is sensed and processed by the biological system generates signals, neural and humoral, which are utilized to control appetite. It follows that any self-imposed or externally applied reduction in the food supply, creating a caloric deficit, will weaken the satiating power of food. One consequence of this will be the failure of food adequately to suppress hunger (the biological drive). The satiety cascade appears to operate as efficiently in obese people as in lean individuals. Therefore, a normal appetite response to reduce calorie intake is evident in obese subjects.

Technically, satiety can be defined as an inhibition of hunger and eating that arises as a consequence of food consumption. It can be distinguished from satiation, which is the process that brings a period of eating to a halt. Consequently, satiation and satiety act conjointly to determine the pattern of eating behaviour and the accompanying profile of motivation. The conscious sensation of hunger is one index of motivation and reflects the strength of satiation and satiety. It is worth remembering that hunger is a biologically useful sensation. It is a nagging, irritating sensation that prompts thoughts of food and reminds us that the body needs energy. The identification and management of hunger are important factors underlying normal appetite function and abnormalities of appetite and body weight.

1.4   Nutrition and satiety

The concept of the satiety cascade implies that foods of varying nutritional composition will engage differently with the mediating

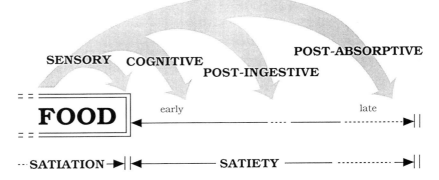

Figure 1.2 Working conceptualization of the satiety cascade illustrating the separation of the processes of satiation and satiety.

processes and will, therefore, exert differing effects upon satiation and satiety. A procedure widely used to assess the action of food on satiety is the preload strategy. Precisely prepared foods (identical in taste and appearance, but varying in energy and/or nutrient composition) can be consumed in the preload. Effects of consumption are then measured over varying periods by visual analogue rating scales (to assess hunger and other sensations), food checklists, accurately monitored test meals and, if necessary, food diaries. The procedure sounds simple, but the conduct of such experiments needs to be governed by a strong methodology to prevent incidental features from interfering with the monitoring process. For example, it is important to prevent the occurrence of any appetite modulating stimuli during the interval between preload and test meal. Such interruption would obviously contaminate the evaluation of the satiating efficiency of the preload.

Using the preload strategy and related procedures, it is possible to assess the satiating power of a wide variety of foods varying in macronutrient composition (Blundell *et al.*, 1988). Indeed, it has been noted that "it would be of great value to have tables showing the energy–satiety ratio of all the common foods to indicate their potential for causing overnutrition" (Heaton, 1981). Foods exerting only a weak effect on satiety would not be expected to provide effective appetite control. There is widespread agreement that the combination and proportions of macronutrients in a food have an important influence on the satiating capacity of a product. Protein appears to be particularly satiating and this has been demonstrated with real foods (e.g. Hill and Blundell, 1990) and with composite formulas (Booth *et al.*, 1970). It is also noticeable that formulations of the trends in macronutrient consumption over the last 100 years have indicated that the proportion of protein in the total energy consumed has remained relatively constant (varying between about 11 and 14 energy percent) even though the availability of protein in the food supply has changed markedly. However, these long term trends indicate that the largest changes have occurred in the consumption of carbohydrate and fat. Whereas, at the turn of the century, carbohydrate intake was about 75% and fat intake about 15% of total energy, today fat consumption constitutes as much as 40% of average energy intake and this increase in fat has occurred simultaneously with a displacement of carbohydrate. In the light of these secular trends much interest is now focused upon low-calorie products which reduce the content of fat and carbohydrate in foods.

It is clear that following consumption of carbohydrates, the digested carbohydrate influences a number of mechanisms involved in satiety. These include glucoreceptors within the gastrointestinal tract (Mei, 1985) that send afferent information via the vagus and splanchnic nerves and glucosensitive cells in the liver, to the nucleus tractus solitarius and hypothalamic regions of the brain which monitor post-absorptive activity of glucose (Oomura, 1988). These mechanisms form the basis of the energostatic control of feeding (Booth, 1972) or what has been called the caloric control of satiety (Blundell and Rogers, 1991). Although sweet carbohydrates induce some positive feedback for eating through oral afferent stimulation, this should be countered by the potent inhibitory action via post-ingestive and post-absorptive mechanisms. Appropriate experiments should demonstrate whether or not this is the case.

One clear finding from these studies is that carbohydrates are efficient appetite suppressants. That is, they contribute markedly to the satiating efficiency of food and exert a potent effect on satiety (Rogers et al., 1988; Rogers and Blundell, 1989). This evidence indicating the potency of metabolized carbohydrate to inhibit appetite is precisely complemented by studies showing that an analogue of glucose, 2-deoxy-D-glucose (which blocks cells' utilization of glucose), actually increased hunger when given to human subjects (Thompson and Campbell, 1977). On the basis of studies on rats, it was argued some years ago that "if the cumulative inhibitory effects of carbohydrate on feeding are indeed energostatic . . . then any substance which can readily be used by the animal to provide energy should produce an appropriate food intake compensation over a period of several hours after loading" (Booth, 1972). Studies have shown that this is exactly the same in humans. A variety of carbohydrates, including glucose, fructose, sucrose and maltodextrins, have rather similar effects when given in a preload. That is, they suppress later intake by an amount roughly equivalent to their caloric value, although the time course of the suppressive action may vary a little based on the rate at which the carbohydrate loads are metabolized.

Only a few studies have systematically investigated the extent to which dietary fat contributes to the satiating power of food. However, there is a widespread belief that high-fat diets are responsible for an elevated energy intake which in turn leads to weight gain through fat deposition. Indeed, there is considerable evidence for a positive relationship between body fatness and the proportion of calories eaten as fat (Dreon et al., 1988; Fricker et al., 1989; Klesges et al., 1992; Romieu et al., 1988).

The actions of carbohydrates and fats on appetite are specially relevant to the potential effects of low-calorie products on dietary habits. Two major classes of low-calorie foods are the high-intensity sweeteners, intended for use as a replacement of sugars, and low-fat products. An evaluation of the physiological and behavioural effects of such foods is important in the light of the current level of overweight in many societies and of the daily intake of fat and carbohydrate.

1.5   Relationship between body weight and use of carbohydrate or high-intensity sweeteners

Commercial advertisements for artificial sweeteners and light products containing artificial sweeteners suggest that the use of these sweeteners help people to attain or maintain a desirable body weight. In theory, this is achieved by the energy reduction which results from the replacement of energetic carbohydrate-based sweeteners by low-calorie intense sweeteners. The key question regarding the use of artificial sweeteners is: do they really help? As with most issues in the field of nutrition the answer is not a simple yes or no. Before discussing any data on the effects of artificial sweeteners it should be emphasized that the use of artificial sweeteners *per se* does not cause weight loss or weight gain. This is because they contain no, or just a little, metabolizable energy.

When evaluating the use of artificial sweeteners, three issues should be considered. The most relevant issue is the relationship between the use of carbohydrate or artificial sweeteners and body weight. As the body weight depends to a large extent on food and energy intake, the second issue concerns the effect of carbohydrate and artificial sweeteners on food and energy intake. The third point of discussion is the effect of carbohydrate sweeteners and artificial sweeteners on feelings of hunger or appetite. The present discussion is limited to the comparison of carbohydrate sweeteners and high-intensity sweeteners.

Whereas in the Middle Ages sugar had a very positive image as a medicine, many people nowadays consider sugar consumption to have negative health effects (Fischler, 1987). Among those negative beliefs is the conviction that the consumption of sugar is fattening (Fischler, 1987). However, it is not clear whether or not this is true. A recent review of the American Food and Drug Administration (FDA) about the health effects of sugar (Glinsmann *et al.*, 1986) came to the conclusion that sugar consumption is not positively related to obesity. There seems to be no evidence that the consumption of sweet carbohydrates is related to body weight. If sugar consumption is not related to body weight, the question arises whether or not a reduction in sugar consumption (achieved by replacement with artificial sweeteners) would result in a lower body weight. This conclusion does not support the idea that the replacement of sugar by artificial sweeteners will be effective in weight control.

The results of a large scale epidemiological study with about 78 000 American women of 50–70 years (Stellman and Garfinkel, 1986) showed that there is a positive relationship between body weight and the prevalence of artificial sweetener use. The same study showed that users of artificial sweeteners gained more weight during one year follow-up than non-users. These data suggest that artificial sweeteners do not help to maintain a desirable body weight. A possible explanation for this result is that the people who used artificial sweeteners are those people who are genetically more prone to obesity compared to the group that do not consume artificial sweeteners. In the same manner, it can also be argued that the people who used artificial sweeteners would have gained even more weight if they had not consumed artificial sweeteners.

1.5.1 Effects on energy intake

Artificial sweeteners uncouple the signal of sweetness with the subsequent flow of energy into the human body. The question with respect to food and energy intake is whether or not the human body detects the difference in energy content and compensates for the missing energy. Several short term and long term studies have been carried out.

1.5.1.1 Repeated consumption. The repeated administration studies can be divided into three reports carried out by Porikos and colleagues, and three other studies carried out by other investigators more recently. Porikos and colleagues (Porikos *et al.*, 1977, 1982; Porikos and Pi-Sunyer, 1984) studied the effects of diets in which the sweet foods contained either sucrose or the high-intensity sweetener aspartame. In these studies, 13 obese and 14 non-obese subjects were placed in metabolic wards and each diet was administered for a 3-day period. Subjects were unaware of the covert experimental manipulation. It was required that the subjects drink a minimum number of soft drinks with either aspartame or sucrose. The question was whether or not subjects would compensate for the energy which was lost following the replacement of sugar by aspartame. The results showed that subjects partly compensated for the missing energy, although the energy intake in the aspartame condition was lower than in the sucrose condition. One striking feature of the results of these careful and well-designed studies is that the initial mean energy consumption was very high. This was during a sucrose condition in each of the three studies. The mean initial energy intakes in these three studies were about 3300, 3800 and 4000 kcal per day, respectively. This suggests a highly palatable and varied diet. One question is whether or not the aspartame-containing diets were equally palatable. Consequently, these studies have failed to resolve unequivocally the question of compensation following substitution of sucrose by aspartame.

Considering the other repeated administration, Tordoff and Alleva (1990) used a within-subjects design with 30 subjects to investigate three experimental conditions. In two conditions subjects were obliged to drink daily for seven days, a volume of 1135 ml soft drink containing either aspartame or fructose. In the third condition there was no mandatory beverage consumption. Daily food and energy intake excluding the energy from the fructose was not different between the fructose and the aspartame condition. Thus, subjects did not compensate for the excess energy of fructose. Subjects had a higher energy intake in the third condition, compared to the aspartame and fructose conditions.

Mattes (1990) investigated the effects of three different breakfasts with equal caloric content (unsweetened, sweetened with sucrose, or sweetened with aspartame) on the energy and macronutrient intake of 24 subjects during five subsequent days. Half of the subjects were informed about the type of sweeteners used. No effects were found for taste or for type of sweetener. However, the subjects who were informed about the type of sweeteners used had a higher mean daily energy intake during the aspartame condition compared to the sucrose condition. The result is important because this condition may reflect the normal use situation.

Kanders et al. (1988) compared the effects of a nine week weight loss programme with sucrose containing products ($n = 30$) with the same weight loss programme with aspartame products ($n = 29$). The women in the aspartame group lost on average 2 kg more than the women in the sucrose group. On the contrary, the men in the aspartame group lost on average 2 kg less than the men in the sucrose group. This result leaves open the question whether aspartame is a useful tool in a weight loss programme.

1.5.1.2 Acute effects.   Most short term studies on the effects of carbohydrate sweeteners and artificial sweeteners on food intake are of the preload–test meal type. In this sort of study subjects receive a preload in which nutritional or sensory variables are manipulated. After such a preload subjects are offered a test meal. A comparison of the energy consumed in the test meal after different preloads gives an indication as to whether subjects compensated for the energy lost by replacing a carbohydrate sweetener by an intense sweetener. It should be noted that the results of these studies depend to a considerable extent on the methodology used. The following is a list of a number of methodological features which may influence the results:

- Type of carbohydrate sweetener used as preload
- Type of artificial sweetener used as preload
- Dose of carbohydrate/artificial sweetener
- Type of food in which sweeteners are used
- Time of the day of study
- Time between preload and test meal
- Composition and type of foods of the test meal
- Characteristics of subjects
- Experimental procedures
- Testing environment.

Considering these variables, it is not surprising that the results of various studies differ. However, some consistent observations emerge. In all but one of the studies (Rolls *et al.*, 1990), subjects had a higher energy intake in a test meal after preloads with artificial sweeteners, than after preloads with carbohydrate sweeteners (Anderson *et al.*, 1989; Birch *et al.*, 1989; Brala and Hagan, 1983 (aspartame vs. sucrose condition); Canty and Chan, 1991; Ho *et al.*, 1990; Rodin, 1990; Rogers and Blundell, 1989; Rogers *et al.* 1988; Rolls *et al.*, 1989). Sometimes these differences were small and statistically insignificant. However, these data indicate that the consumption of sweeteners with carbohydrate energy suppress later intake more than sweetness alone or with less energy. Usually only partial compensation is observed.

1.5.2   Effects on subjective feelings of hunger

In general it can be stated that the ingestion of food leads to a reduction in subjective appetite. The degree to which this reduction takes place depends on the properties of food. Weight, volume, taste, structure and energy, and macronutrient content are all properties which have an effect on appetite. The main difference between carbohydrate sweeteners and artificial sweeteners lies in the energy content, apart from the difference in bulk. Therefore, it seems plausible to assume that energy contributes to satiety, which would lead to the expectation that carbohydrate sweeteners are more satiating than artificial sweeteners. However, the data of studies comparing the effects of both types of sweeteners on appetite are not very consistent.

In the studies of Anderson *et al.* (1989), Canty and Chan (1991), Rogers and Blundell (1989), and Rogers *et al.* (1988), hunger ratings were higher after loads with artificial sweeteners than after loads with carbohydrate sweeteners. In the studies of Anderson *et al.* (1989) and Canty and Chan (1991) the differences were not significant. Rolls *et al.* (1989, 1990) did not find any differences between the effects of carbohydrate sweeteners and artificial sweeteners. However, methodological factors are particularly important here since the subjective sensations of hunger could be disrupted by psychological or physiological interference between the preload and the test meal. Accordingly, it should be noted that in those studies which incorporated an estimation of sensory specific satiety it is customary to give nine taste samples on four occasions during this interval. This procedure is likely to contaminate the process mediating the effect of the preload upon the test meal. Such contamination would invalidate not only the subjective ratings of hunger, but also the food consumption in the test meal.

1.5.3   Overview

High intensity sweeteners: do they really help? Considering the empirical evidence, there is no simple yes or no to this question. On the one hand, there is no evidence for a positive relationship between sugar use and body weight. This raises the question of whether a reduction in sugar use by replacement with artificial sweetener would lead to reduction in body weight. On the other hand, there is some evidence for a positive relationship between artificial sweetener use and body weight, although this relationship may be confounded by a genetic predisposition for obesity.

Repeated consumption studies on the effect of carbohydrate sweeteners and body weight on energy intake show mixed results. In some studies there is some caloric compensation in the artificial sweetener condition; in other studies there is not. Most acute preload–test meal studies show that subjects eat more after a preload with an artificial sweetener than after a preload with carbohydrate sweetener. However, compensation was rarely complete. The data on the effects of carbohydrate and artificial sweeteners on subjective feelings of appetite also show mixed results. In some studies subjects report less hunger after carbohydrate sweeteners than after artificial sweeteners. In other studies both types of sweeteners have similar effects on hunger. The importance of methodological factors should be kept in mind when evaluating these effects.

The fact that the results of various studies differ is not surprising considering the complexity of the issue. There are numerous experimental factors which can have a substantial effect on the results. The same is true for the effect of artificial sweetener use on body weight in daily life. When do people use artificial sweeteners, and in what type of products? How much do they use them? For what purpose do they use them? What do people think that artificial sweeteners do for them? Advertisements suggest that the consumption of artificial sweeteners will make people slim automatically. This is of course not true. When, for instance, people replace sugar in coffee with artificial sweeteners, do they believe they therefore have a licence to take a cookie or cake in addition? It seems that the effect of artificial sweetener use on body weight in real life situations depends to a large extent on these factors.

It can be concluded that the effect of high-intensity sweeteners on appetite and body weight will depend on the interaction between physiological and psychological factors. The effects of sweeteners *per se* and energy *per se* on the body will be influenced by the subject's cognitions regarding the likely effect of the food product and the extent to which this product is being used judiciously within a system of dietary control. High-intensity sweeteners do not automatically lead to weight loss, but if used sensibly within a disciplined regime they could be useful.

1.6 Dietary fat and appetite control

It is widely recognized that the consumption of dietary fat in many societies is unacceptably high. For example, a recent survey carried out by the Office of Population Consensus and Surveys (OPCS, 1990) between the years 1986 and 1987 revealed that the average daily fat intake for British men was 102 g and that this constituted 40.2% of total food energy. For women the figures were 73 g and 40.3%. Similar data have been reported in the USA (Cronin and Shaw, 1988). These amounts are considerably in excess of the 35% of food energy recommended in the reports of a number of advisory bodies (for example, NACNE, 1983). What do these data tell us about the relationship between dietary fat and appetite control?

In the scientific study of the control of food intake certain classical hypotheses have attempted to account for the modulation of appetite through the monitoring of dietary commodities or some physiological factor related to energy intake. These propositions are known as the glucostatic (Mayer, 1953), aminostatic (Mellinkoff *et al.*, 1955) and lipostatic (Kennedy, 1953) hypotheses. There is good evidence for the existence of glucosensitive cells and glucoreceptor neurons in liver, nucleus of the tractus solitarius and the hypothalamus (Oomura, 1988). Receptors for amino acids exist in the gastrointestinal tract and their activity is relayed to the solitary tract via the afferent vagus (Mei, 1985) The lipostatic hypothesis is not well supported. The phenomenon of diet induced obesity suggests that excessive energy intake leading to an increase in body fat stores does not exert an inhibitory action on food intake (Rogers and Blundell, 1984; Sclafani, 1984). Moreover, in obese people the amount of body fat does not appear to apply a braking action on the biological drive of appetite. Indeed, because of the increase in resting metabolic rate due to increased body size, energy intake in the obese is elevated in order to maintain energy balance. Although various chemicals have been mentioned as candidates to signal the amount of body fat (e.g. fat mobilizing substance, adipsin), such a potential role does not appear to be supported by evidence.

However, even though adipose tissue itself does not provide a signal for appetite, the consumption of dietary fat may influence the expression of appetite. This could occur in at least two ways. First, by the energy or nutritional value of the consumed fat being monitored (by specialized receptors or metabolic processes) and this information used to adjust the selected volitional intake of fat. Second, by the consumed fat activating post-ingestive mechanisms which exert an immediate inhibitory action on intake. An example of the first mechanism would be the release of the co-lipase activating enzyme known as enterostatin (Erlanson-Albertson and Larsson, 1988), whilst the second mechanism is represented by the phenomenon of fat-stimulated release of cholecystokinin (Greenberg *et al.*, 1989). Through these, and possibly other mechanisms, the consumption of fat could exert an inhibitory action upon overall energy intake or the selective intake of fat.

1.6.1 Experimental manipulations

It is worth noting that there may be differing responses to the overconsumption or underconsumption of fat. These have been termed the fat-minus and the fat-plus manipulations (Blundell and Burley, 1991) and experimental designs should investigate both of these phenomena. There is some evidence that the compensation for a reduction in dietary fat energy is incomplete in normal weight subjects (Hill *et al.*, 1987) or virtually absent in overweight subjects (Lissner *et al.*, 1987). Other studies have indicated that meals with a high fat:carbohydrate ratio suppress hunger to a lesser degree than meals with a low fat:carbohydrate ratio (Van Amelsvoort *et al.*, 1989). In addition, it has been reported that intravenous infusion of a fixed amount of energy provided as fat, suppressed subsequent oral energy intake to a lesser degree than did an equi-caloric infusion of amino acids and carbohydrate (Friedman, 1990). In turn it is known that a dietary intake high in fat (reflected by the food quotient, FQ) is strongly correlated with weight gain (Tremblay *et al.*, 1989). Moreover, Lissner and colleagues have demonstrated that subjects under-ate when forced to eat low-fat foods (high FQ diets) for three weeks and over-ate (relative to a medium-fat diet) when obliged to consume from an assortment of high-fat foods (low FQ diet) (Lissner *et al.*, 1987). During the period on the high-fat diets subjects consumed an additional 362 kcal per day (surfeit of 15.4%) compared to the medium diet and gained an average of 0.32 kg body weight. The results of these studies suggest two possibilities. First that people are actively seeking dietary fat and when offered an opportunity they actively ingest the commodity thereby increasing caloric intake. Second that people exposed to a high-fat diet display a passive tendency to overconsume calories. In both cases the excessive energy intake does not appear to be subjected to any potent inhibitory action from the monitoring of the ingested fat. If this is the case and if withdrawing dietary fat induces a less intense caloric compensation than other energy-yielding dietary constituents, then the replacement of dietary fat by a non-absorbable fat substitute would be a useful strategy to reduce overall caloric or fat intake.

At the present time only a limited number of studies are available as a basis for deducing the relationship between dietary fat and the control of appetite. However, considering the concept of satiating efficiency together with the preload or meal supplementation design, the following conclusions can be drawn.

— Dietary supplements of 36–40 g of fat at a breakfast meal do not significantly adjust the satiating power of food or lead to any compensation in intake for at least eight hours after consumption. Moreover, in most of these studies the extra fat consumed at breakfast augments the total daily energy intake (Cotton *et al.*, 1992).

— Supplements of carbohydrate and fat differ in their measured effects on satiety. Carbohydrate produces an intensification of satiety which is clearly detectable for a limited period after consumption. The concept of the post-ingestive window can be used to signify the importance of the time course of satiety.

However, as with the assesment of effects of intense sweeteners, the experimental results of studies on fat are not in good agreement with each other. A number of studies have reported that there appears to be good caloric compensation for the covert manipulation of fat in normal foods. Once again these differences draw attention to methodological variables in experimental designs which may influence the measured actions of any manipulation.

1.6.2 Satiation and satiety in response to fat

One conceptual limitation of experimental designs may concern the satiating efficiency of food; this notion invites researchers experimentally to manipulate fat and to measure the consequences of consuming a predetermined quantity. An alternative strategy is to reverse the direction of experimental causality and to measure effects upon fat intake rather than the effects of fat consumption. In practice, this means evaluating the effects of psychological or physiological manipulation on the consumption of high-fat foods (compared with low-fat foods). This procedure will measure the compensatory response of fat rather than its satiating power. Of course under circumstances of natural intake both processes take place concurrently and it is only for theoretical clarity and experimental convenience that they are treated separately. Consequently, explanations of the relationship between dietary fat and appetite require experimental investigation of satiating power and compensatory response. In turn, this will disclose the action of fat upon satiation (within meals) and satiety (after meals).

An experimental design to implement this objective is set out in Figure 1.3. The objective of the design is to assess the capacity of high-fat or high-carbohydrate foods to lead to overconsumption by an action on either satiation, satiety or both. Unlike many studies in this area of research, the levels of intake of fat and carbohydrate were voluntarily set by each subject's own consumption rather than being externally manipulated by the experimenter. Therefore, the relative effects of these two macronutrients on satiation and satiety can be compared.

Table 1.1 indicates that exposure to high-fat foods generates a large energy intake within meals. That is, fat has a weak effect on satiation. In addition the suppressive action of this large energy intake on later consumption is disproportionately small. That is, fat has a relatively weak effect on satiety when large amounts are consumed. However, it could be

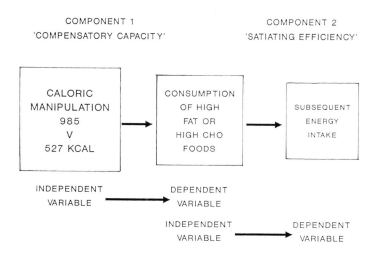

Figure 1.3 Experimental design for the simultaneous evaluation of foods on satiation (meal size) and satiety (post-meal effects).

argued that this large intake of calories on exposure to high-fat foods would lead to caloric compensation much later, possibly during the following day when subjects may consume fewer calories to balance the excess previously taken in. However, energy intake on the following day (calculated from food diary records) did not show evidence of caloric adjustment. Average energy intakes were 1800 and 1556 kcal, respectively, after the high-fat and high-carbohydrate meals. Though not statistically significant the direction of this difference is opposite to that predicted on the expectation of caloric compensation.

1.6.3 Dietary fat and appetite—is there a paradox?

Considering the literature on the relationship between dietary fat, food intake and body weight, there may appear to be a paradox. On the one hand, a number of studies indicate a positive correlation between body fat

Table 1.1 Comparison of the effects of high-fat and high-carbohydrate foods on energy intake within a meal (satiation) and following a meal (satiety)

Mean intake at dinner (kcal)—*satiation effect*	
High fat	High CHO
1336	677
Mean post-dinner intake (kcal)—*satiety effect*	
310	391

(or body mass index) and the proportion of fat in the diet. In addition when subjects are exposed to high-fat diets they overconsume energy and usually gain weight. On the other hand, a number of studies which have covertly manipulated fat in foods have apparently found that fat can induce a reasonable degree of satiety. How is it that fat can induce normal satiety (control over appetite) yet people can overconsume fat and gain weight? If fat were exerting a control over appetite through the processes of satiety, then overconsumption should not be possible. There are two possible explanations. One is that people deliberately override their own satiety signals and voluntarily overconsume fat. Another is that the major effect of fat is to weaken satiation (and allow very large meals to be consumed). Since satiation is not normally measured in short term studies on the effect of fat on appetite, the disclosure of this action can help to explain the apparent paradox. Satiation, rather than satiety may be the most important process in allowing us to understand the effect of dietary fat upon food intake and body weight.

1.7 Low-calorie products—physiological responses

The low-calorie products considered in this chapter have been those relating to dietary carbohydrate and fat. The effects of foods which are intended to allow people to lower the consumption of these nutrients will obviously depend upon the effects of the nutrients themselves and the way in which they are used by the body. The evidence reported above indicates that the physiological responses of the body to fat and carbohydrate are different. One influential theoretical formulation which helps us to understand the relationship between the physiological and behavioural effects of carbohydrate and fat is the concept of nutrient balance (e.g. Flatt *et al.*, 1988). In brief this concept is based on the observation that the dietary intakes of carbohydrate and protein are tightly coupled to their rates of utilization in the body whilst the body's capacity to store these nutrients is limited. On the other hand dietary fat intake is not closely related to the rate of fat oxidation (although this depends on genetic susceptibility) and the capacity for fat storage in the body is large. Therefore, a high intake of fat would not normally lead to an increase in fat utilization, but would be stored. On the other hand an increased intake of carbohydrate would tend to drive up carbohydrate oxidation since storage capacity is in any case limited. Moreover, it appears that the *de novo* conversion of carbohydrate to fat is normally a very weak pathway (Acheson *et al.*, 1988). These ideas and data have led to the conclusion that

> Fat calories represent the only candidate for a sufficient chronic energy imbalance to cause obesity, implying that in addition to an increase in exercise

and restriction of total calories (both manoeuvres stimulating fat oxidation), a simple reduction in fat intake will lead to weight loss. This has now been demonstrated in several short and medium term studies of low-fat, *ad libitum* diets (Kendall *et al.*, 1991). This approach cannot be expected to produce the rapid weight loss commonly seen in restricted energy diets of 800–1200 kcal per day, but could serve as the central strategy for the prevention and treatment of obesity at the individual and population levels. A crucial point to this approach is whether the previously obese patient is able consciously and permanently to reduce the amount of fat in the diet despite a natural (most likely genetic) preference for fatty food. Encouraging the food industry to produce and promote low-fat products, and educating consumers to choose those products, are probably the best options for population-wide dietary changes. (Ravussin and Swinburn, 1992, p. 408.)

Accordingly, considering the relevance of low-calorie products for the control of body weight, the difference in potency of carbohydrate and fat substitutes seems clear.

1.8   Low-calorie products—psychological responses

The way in which dietary carbohydrate and fat influence the psychological sensations associated with the motivation to eat have been set out above. The situation can be summarized by stating that the feeling of hunger appears to be much more responsive to changes in the supply of carbohydrates than of fat. This is in keeping with the responses induced in food consumption. Such responses are observed best under scientifically controlled conditions when the nutrient manipulations are disguised. Hence the results tend to represent the unconditioned biological response. However, in more natural situations outside of laboratories or controlled studies, low-calorie products are usually consumed when their nutrient content is known to the consumer. Often a person would know that they are eating a low-carbohydrate or a reduced-fat product. Under these circumstances the influence of cognitions or beliefs would begin to affect motivation and eating. Short term studies which have investigated this have frequently found that, after consuming a product for which the nutritional content and their beliefs about the nutritional content have been manipulated, people subsequently eat in accordance with their beliefs or expectations. In real life this may mean that people knowingly eating low-calorie foods may eat more later thereby allowing themselves to 'make up' for the calories they 'know' they have lost.

One further issue concerns the effect of nutrients on psychological features not associated with the motivation to eat. These include changes in mood, feelings of well being and cognitive and physical performance (Levine and Krahn, 1988). This area has not yet been extensively researched, but it is fully expected that changes in the dietary intake of carbohydrates and fats due to the consumption of low-calorie products will give rise to changes in psychological states. Some changes may be beneficial and lead to enhanced feelings of well being and performance whilst other adjustments may be detrimental. The evaluation of such changes may pose dilemmas. For example, when it is reported that consumption of a meal rich in a particular nutrient leads to increased lethargy (e.g. Spring *et al.*, 1989) should this be interpreted positively or negatively? On the one hand a feeling of lethargy may be a component of that soothing, tranquilizing quality which is percieved as a pleasant consequence of eating. On the other hand, it could be interpreted as an irritating impediment to active work. One important issue requiring attention is the assessment of the psychological changes induced by long term lipid lowering diets.

1.9 Summary

This review has focused on the effects of low-calorie products involving carbohydrate and fat and their relevance for the control of body weight. The evidence concerning high-intensity sweeteners, carbohydrate substitution and dietary fat on appetite and body weight has been assessed. On the basis of this assessment recommendations about the judicious use of low-calorie products to exert a control over appetite, to induce weight loss or to prevent weight gain can be made. The key to understanding this issue seems to rest upon the different and separate roles played by carbohydrate and fat in the biological and behavioural responses involved in energy balance. However, such biological responses may mean only a little unless attitudes to food products and habitual food preferences can be modified. In addition, cognitions or expectations about the effects of foods certainly modulate the physiological effects. Consequently, the development of low-calorie products poses a continuing challenge for behavioural scientists. Nutritional technology can produce products with an appropriate structure and with appealing sensory qualities which should be acceptable to consumers. Can such products overcome the physiological and psychological defences in order to allow people to consume a more healthy diet? Some indicators are already known, others remain to be discovered, but urgently.

References

Acheson, K.J., Schultz, Y., Bessard, T., Anantharaman, K., Flatt, J.P. and Jequier, E. (1988) Glycogen storage capacity and *de novo* lipogenesis during massive carbohydrate overfeeding in man. *Am. J. Clin. Nutr.*, **48**, 240–247.

Anderson, G.H., Saravis, S., Schacher, R., Zlokin, S. and Leiter, L.A. (1989) Aspartame: Effect on lunch time food intake, appetite and hedonic response in children. *Appetite*, **13**, 93–103.

Birch, L.L., McPhee, L. and Sullivan, S. (1989) Children's food intake following drinks sweetened with sucrose or aspartame: time course effects. *Physiol. Behav.*, **45**, 387–395.

Blundell, J.E. and Burley, V.J. (1991) Evaluation of the satiating power of dietary fat in man. In: *Progress in Obesity Research 1990.* (Eds Y. Oomura, S. Baba and T. Shimazu). J. Libbey and Sons, London, pp. 453–457.

Blundell, J.E. and Hill, A.J. (1986) Biopsychological interactions underlying the study and treatment of obesity. In: *The Psychosomatic Approach: Contemporary Practise in Whole Person Care* (eds M.J. Christie and P.G. Mellett). Wiley, Chichester, pp. 115–138.

Blundell, J.E. and Rogers, P.J. (1991) Hunger, hedonics and the control of satiation and satiety. In: *Chemical Senses, Vol.4: Appetite and Nutrition* (eds M. Friedman and M. Kare). Marcel Dekker, New York, pp. 127–148.

Blundell, J.E., Rogers, P.J. and Hill, A.J. (1987) Evaluating the satiating power of foods: implications for acceptance and consumption. In: *Chemical Composition and Sensory Properties of Food and their Influence on Nutrition* (ed. J. Solms). Academic Press, London, pp. 205–219.

Blundell, J.E., Hill, A.J. and Rogers, P.J. (1988) Hunger and the satiety cascade – their importance for food acceptance in the late 20th century. In: *Food Acceptability* (ed. D.M.H. Thompson). Elsevier Applied Science, London and New York, pp. 233–250.

Booth, D.A. (1972) Postabsorptively induced suppression of appetite and the energostatic control of feeding. *Physiol. Behav.*, **9**, 199–202.

Booth, D.A., Chase, A. and Campbell, A.T. (1970) Relative effectiveness of protein in the late stages of appetite suppression in man. *Physiol. Behav.*, **5**, 1299–1302.

Bouchard, C. (1985) Inheritance of fat distribution and adipose tissue metabolism. In: *Metabolic Complications of Human Obesities* (eds J. Vague, P. Bjovntorp, B. Guy-Grand, M. Rebuffe-Scrive and P. Vague). Excerpta Medica, Amsterdam, pp. 87–96.

Brala, P.M. and Hagen, R.L. (1983) Effects of sweetness perception and caloric value of a preload on short term intake. *Physiol. Behav.*, **30**, 1–10.

Canty, D.J. and Chan, M.M. (1991) Effects of consumption of caloric vs. non-caloric sweet drinks in indices of hunger and food consumption in normal adults. *Am. J. Clin. Nutr.*, **53**, 1159–1164.

Cronin, F.J. and Shaw, A.M. (1988) Summary of dietary recommendations for healthy Americans. *Nutrition Today*, November/December, 26–34.

Dreon, D.M., Frey-Hewitt, B., Ellsworth, N., Williams, P.T., Terry, R.B. and Wood P.D. (1988) Dietary fat: carbohydrate ratio and obesity in middle aged men. *Am. J. Clin. Nutr.*, **47**, 995–1000.

Erlanson-Albertsson, C. and Larsson, A. (1988) The activation peptide of pancreatic procolipase decreases food intake in rats. *Regulatory Peptides*, **22**, 325–331.

Fischler, C. (1987) Attitudes towards sugar in historical and social perspective. In: *Sweetness* (ed. J. Dobbing). Springer-Verlag; London, pp. 83–98.

Flatt, J.P., Ravussin, E., Acheson, K.J. and Jequier, E. (1988) Effects of dietary fat on postprandial substrate oxidation and on carbohydrate and fat balances. *J. Clin. Invest*, **7**, 1019–1024.

Fricker, J., Fumeron, F., Didier, C. and Apfelbaum, M. (1989) A positive correlation between energy intake and body mass index in a population of 1312 overweight subjects. *Internat. J. Obesity*, 663–681.

Friedman, M.I. (1990) Body fat and the metabolic control of food intake. *Int. J. Obesity*, **14** (suppl. 3), 53–67.

Garrow, J.S. (1992) Treatment of obesity. *The Lancet*, **340**, 409–413.

Glinsmann, W.H., Irausquin, H.M. and Park, Y.K. (1986) Evaluation of health aspects of sugars contained in carbohydrate sweeteners: report of sugar task force. *J. Nutr.*, **116** (November suppl.), S1–S216 (see pp. S106 and S107).

Greenberg, D., Torres, N.I., Smith, G.P. and Gibbs, J. (1989) The satiating effect of fats is attenuated by the cholecystokinin antagonist Lorglumide. *Ann. N.Y. Acad. Sci.*, **575**, 517–520.

Heaton, K.W. (1981) Dietary fibre and energy intake. In: *Regulators of Intestinal Absorption in Obesity, Diabetes and Nutrition* (eds P. Berchtold, A. Cairella, A. Jacobelli and V. Silvano). Societa Editrice Universo, Roma, pp.238–294.

Hill, A.J. and Blundell, J.E. (1990) Sensitivity of the appetite control system in obese subjects to nutritional and serotoninergic challenges. *Int. J. Obesity*, **14**, 219–233.

Hill, A.J., Leathwood, P.J. and Blundell, J.E. (1987) Some evidence for short term caloric compensation in normal weight human subjects: The effects of high and low energy meals on hunger, food preference and food intake. *Human Nutr. Appl. Nutr.*, **41A**, 244–257.

Ho, E.E., Liszt, A. and Pudel, V. (1990) The effects of energy content and sweet taste on food consumption in restrained and non-restrained eaters. *J. Am. Diet. Assoc.*, **90**, 1223–1228.

Kanders, B.S., Lavine, P.T., Kowalchuck, M.B., Greenberg, I. and Blackburn, G.L. (1988) An evaluation of the effect of aspartame on weight loss. *Appetite*, **11** suppl, 73–84.

Kendall, A., Levitsky, D.A., Strupp, B.J. and Lissner, L. (1991) Weight loss on a low-fat diet:consequence of the imprecision of the control of food intake in humans. *Am. J. Clin. Nutr.*, **53**, 112–1129.

Kennedy, G.C. (1953) The role of depot fat in the hypothalamic control of food intake in the rat. *Proc. Roy. Soc. London, Ser. B.*, **140**, 578–592.

Kissileff, H.R. (1984) Satiating efficiency and a strategy for conducting food loading experiments. *Neurosci. Biobehav. Rev.*, **8**, 129–135.

Klesges, R.C., Klesges, L.M., Haddock, C.K. and Eck, L.H. (1992) A longitudinal analysis of the impact of dietary intake and physical activity on weight change in adults. *Am. J. Clin. Nutr.*, **55**, 818–822.

Levine, A.S. and Krahn, D.D.(1988) Food and behaviour. In: *Nutritional Modulation of Neural Function* (eds J.E. Morley, M.D. Sterman and J.H. Walsh). Academic Press, San Diego, pp. 233–250.

Lissner, L., Levitsky, D.A., Strupp, B.J., Kackwarf, H. and Roe, D.A. (1987) Dietary fat and the regulation of energy intake in human subjects. *Am. J. Clin. Nutr.*, **46**, 886–892.

Mattes, R. (1990) Effects of aspartame and sucrose on hunger and energy intake in humans. *Physiol. Behav.*, **47**, 1037–1044.

Mayer, J. (1953) Glucostatic mechanism of the regulation of food intake. *New England J. Medicine*, **249**, 13–16.

Mei, N. (1985) Intestinal chemosensitivity. *Physiol. Rev.*, **65**, 211–237.

Mellinkoff, S.M., Frankland, M., Boyle, D. and Greipel, M. (1955) The effect of amino acid administration upon the blood sugar concentration. *Stanford Med. Bull.*, **13**; 117–124.

NACNE (National Advisory Committee for Nutrition Education) (1983). *Proposals for Nutrition Guidelines for Health Education in Britain*. Health Education Council, London.

Oomura, Y. (1988) Chemical and neuronal control of feeding motivation. *Physiol. Behav.*, **44**, 555–560.

OPCS (Office of Population Censuses and Surveys) (1990). *The Dietary and Nutritional Survey of British Adults*. HMSO, London, 393 pp.

Porikos, K.P. and Pi-Sunyer F.X. (1984) Regulation of food intake in human obesity: studies with caloric dilution. *Clin. Endocrinol. Metab.*, **13**, 547–561

Porikos, K.P., Booth, G. and Van Itallie, T.B. (1977) Effect of covert nutritive dilution on the spontaneous food intake of obese individuals: a pilot study. *Am. J. Clin. Nutr.*, **30**, 1638–1644.

Porikos, K.P., Hesser, M.F. and Van Itallie, T.B. (1982) Caloric regulation in normal-weight men maintained on a palatable diet of conventional foods. *Physiol. Behav.*, **29**, 293–300

Prentice, A.M., Black, A.E., Murgatroyd, P.R., Goldberg, G.R. and Coward, W.A. (1989) Metabolism or appetite: Questions of energy balance with particular reference to obesity. *J. Human Nut. Dietetics*, **2**, 95–104

Ravussin, E. and Swinburn, B.A. (1992) Pathophysiology of obesity. *The Lancet*, **340**, 404–408.

Richter, C.P. (1943) Total self-regulatory functions in animals and human beings. *Harvey Lecture Series*, **38**, 63–103.

Rodin, J. (1990) Comparative effects of fructose, aspartame, glucose and water preloads on calorie and macronutrient intake. *Am. J. Clin. Nutr.*, **51**, 428–435.

Rogers, P.J. and Blundell, J.E. (1984) Meal patterns and food selection during the development of obesity in rats fed a cafeteria diet. *Neurosci. Biobehav. Rev.*, **8**, 441–453.

Rogers, P.J. and Blundell, J.E. (1989) Separating the action of sweetness and calories: Effects of saccharin and carbohydrates on hunger and food intake in human subjects. *Physiol Behav.*, **45**, 1093–1099

Rogers, P.J., Carlyle, J.A., Hill, A.J. and Blundell, J.E. (1988) Uncoupling sweet taste and calories: Comparison of the effects of glucose and three intense sweeteners on hunger and food intake. *Physiol. Behav.*, **43**, 547–52

Rolls, B.J., Jacobs, L., Laster, L. and Summerfelt, A. (1989) Hunger and food intake following consumption of low-calorie foods. *Appetite*, **13**, 115–27.

Rolls, B.J., Kim, S. and Fedoroff, I.C. (1990) Effects of drinks sweetened with sucrose or aspartame on hunger, thirst and food intake in man. *Physiol. Behav.*, **48**, 19–26.

Romieu, I., Willett, W., Stampfer, M.J., Colditz, G.A., Sampson, L., Rosner, B., Hennekens, C.H. and Speizer, F.E. (1988) Energy intake and other determinants of relative weight. *Am J. Clin. Nutr.*, **47**, 400–412

Sclafani, A. (1984) Animal models of obesity: classification and characterisation. *Int. J. Obesity*, **8**, 491–508.

Spring, B, Chiodo, J., Harden, M., Bourgedis, M.J., Mason, J.D. and Lutherer, L. (1989) Psychobiological effects of carbohydrates. *J. Clin. Psychiatry*, **5**, 27–33

Stellman, S.D. and Garfinkel, L. (1986) Artificial sweetener use and one-year weight change among women. *Preventive Medicine*, **15**, 195–201.

Thompson, D.A. and Campbell, R.G. (1977) Hunger in humans induced by 2-deoxy-d glucose: glucoprivic control of taste preference and food intake. *Science*, **198**, 1065–1068.

Tordoff, M.G. and Alleva, A.M. (1990) Effect of drinking soda sweetened with aspartame or high-fructose corn syrup on food intake and body weight. *Am J. Clin. Nutr.*, **51**, 963–996.

Tremblay, A., Plourde, G., Despres, J.P. and Bouchard, C. (1989) Impact of dietary fat content and fat oxidation and energy intake in humans. *Am. J. Clin. Nutr.*, **49**, 799–805.

Van Amelsvoort, J.M.M., Van Stratum, P., Kraal, J.H., Lussenburg, R.N. and Houtsmuller, U.M.T. (1989) Effects of varying the carbohydrate fat ratio in a hot lunch on postprandial variables in male volunteers. *Br. J. Nutr.*, **61**, 267–283.

2 Regulatory aspects of low-calorie food

G. URQUHART and S.V. MOLINARY

2.1 Introduction

Low-calorie food, for the purposes of this chapter, is food which has had its calorific value reduced by the replacement of a caloric component by a non-caloric additive or by a less energy dense nutrient. Low-calorie food is subject to regulatory constraints in the following areas:

1. Controls on the ingredients: The additives used in low-calorie foods, and in other foods, are subject to extensive safety assessments and restrictions on their levels of use.
2. Controls on the composition of low-calorie foods: These are aimed at protecting the nutritional integrity of the food and are particularly relevant where fat is the component which has been substituted, due to the complex role played by fat in nutrition.
3. Controls on novel foods: Particularly those where a raw material is being put to a novel use.
4. Controls on the labelling of low-calorie foods: Aimed at preventing misleading claims, ensuring the provision of nutritional information to the consumer and medical information to special patient groups.

These controls will be looked at in more detail below. However, it should be noted that the legislation covering all the above aspects is in an extremely dynamic state of change at the time of writing, particularly in the EC and in the USA.

2.2 Regulatory bodies

When considering the regulatory aspects of low-calorie foods the role of those international and national authorities responsible for developing food legislation must be considered.

2.2.1 International bodies

In 1963 the Food and Agriculture Organization of the United Nations and the World Health Organisation established the FAO/WHO Codex Alimentarius Commission. Its role was to examine food standards on an international basis. One of the many subsidiary bodies established by the Commission since its inception is the Joint FAO/WHO Expert Committee on Food Additives (JECFA) whose role it is to advise the Commission, via the Codex Committee on Food Additives, on the safety of food additives and contaminants in food by publishing maximum levels of food additives and contaminants permitted for use in specific food items (acceptable daily intake, ADI) as well as specifications and toxicological monographs on substances they have considered.

The recommendations of JECFA are not mandatory on national governments, but they are influential in determining legislation at a national level. For example, the Swedish Food Regulations state "If the Food and Agriculture Organization of the United Nations (FAO) and the World Health Organization (WHO) have issued recommendations for the identity and purity of a food additive, the standards in those recommendations shall be complied with." (SLV FS 1991: 7.)

In Europe, the policy making process in terms of food legislation is increasingly being carried out by the bodies within the infrastructure of the European Community rather than by the regulatory bodies of the individual member states. The most important of these bodies is the Scientific Committee on Food (SCF) which was established by the European Commission in 1974. The SCF consists of highly qualified scientists appointed from the various member states from such fields as medicine, nutrition, toxicology, chemistry and biology. At the request of the Commission, the SCF will give its opinion on any problem concerning public health which may result from the consumption of food. The Commission then frames legislation based on the advice given by the SCF, so, unlike JECFA, opinions expressed by the SCF have a direct effect on EC legislation.

By 1993 it is hoped that all food legislation within the EC will have been harmonized. It is unclear at this stage exactly what role the individual member states' regulatory bodies will play after this date. However, there are proposals that national bodies should cooperate in the preparation of the scientific assessments necessary for the provision of opinions by the SCF (COM (92) 128 final–SYN 332).

2.2.2 National bodies

There is a strong trend towards harmonizing national food legislation with that of the EC, not only within the European Community but also in the rest of Europe and in Scandinavia, particularly in those countries who are aspiring to membership of the Community. It seems likely, therefore, that the influence of even the previously well resourced and respected authorities such as the Swedish National Food Administration will be gradually eclipsed by the SCF after 1993.

Outside Europe, there are authorities which are considered as 'benchmark' regulators in terms of both the resources they have at their disposal and the scientific credibility of their opinions. The most influential of these is the United States' Center for Food Safety and Nutrition (CFSAN) of the

Food and Drug Administration (FDA). However, the opinions of the Health Protection Branch of Canada (HPB), the National Food Authority (NFA) of Australia and the Food Sanitation Research Council which advises the Life Hygiene Bureau of the Ministry of Health and Welfare in Japan, are all influential in the international forum.

Although all countries in the world have their own unique systems of food legislation with various levels of sophistication, there has been a strong trend in recent years to harmonize food legislation on a worldwide basis. This is exemplified by tripartite meetings between the United States, Canada and the United Kingdom which are held on an informal basis to discuss food safety matters.

2.3   Controls on the components of low-calorie foods

Low-calorie food can be considered as being made up of two components, food ingredients (carbohydrate, fat and protein) and additives. The latter, which include bulking agents, fat substitutes and high-intensity sweeteners, must meet stringent safety requirements.

2.3.1   Additives

The intentional addition of non-nutritive additives to food must not compromise the wholesomeness of that food. In the European Community the criteria used in approving a food additive are:

- that there can be demonstrated a reasonable technological need for the additive and the purpose for which it is used cannot be achieved by other means which are economically and technologically practicable;
- that the additive presents no hazard to the health of the consumer at the level of use proposed, so far as can be judged on the scientific evidence available;
- that the additive does not mislead the consumer.(89/107/EEC.)

The United States do not have a requirement that a rigorous case for technological need be made as does the European Community. Their criteria are that the the additive must be safe, function in the purported manner, and will not result in the consumer being misled or lead to adulteration. (21 CFR 409.)

2.3.2   Definition of additives

A food additive is defined by the EC (89/107/EEC) as

any substance not normally consumed as a food in itself and not normally used as a characteristic ingredient of food whether or not it has nutritive value, the intentional addition of which to food for a technological purpose in the manufacture, processing or storage of such food results, or may be reasonably expected to result in it or its by-products becoming directly or indirectly a component of such foods.

The United States' definition of food additive is

> any substance the intended use of which results or may reasonably be expected to result, directly or indirectly, in its becoming a component or otherwise affecting the characteristic of any food. . . . (21 CFR170.3.)

This definition is broader than the EC one and incorporates indirect additives such as components of packaging material.

The United States, uniquely, has two categories of substances known as GRAS (Generally Recognized As Safe) substances and 'prior sanction' substances. These are excluded from classification as additives even if they fall into the definition above. A GRAS substance is a substance

> generally recognized, amongst experts qualified by scientific training and experience to evaluate its safety, as having been adequately shown through scientific procedures (or, in the case of a substance used in food prior to January 1, 1958, through either scientific procedures or experience based on common use in food) to be safe under the conditions of its intended use:. . . . (FFDCA 201.)

The parenthetical section of the above definition refers to substances which are entitled to prior sanction status, that is, substances such as sodium nitrate as a preservative in luncheon meats which the FDA or the US Department of Agriculture had determined as safe prior to 1958.

Establishing a GRAS status for a substance requires a similar amount of data to that required for a food additive petition. However, in the case of a GRAS substance the data are taken from existing scientific literature whereas with a new additive most data have not been published.

For historical reasons Japan separates synthetically made food additives, known as 'chemical synthetic compounds,' from 'natural' additives (FAA, 1981). Natural additives, for example thaumatin, are subject to different restrictions from synthetic additives.

2.3.3 Safety assessment of additives

The potential for toxicity, if any, of a food additive must be weighed against its potential consumer exposure. This is the principle of risk assessment.

Any substance, given in large enough amounts can have a deleterious effect on animals. In the safety evaluation of a food additive an attempt is made to quantify this potential for toxicity so that the quantity of that additive consumed is controlled in order to give "an adequate margin of safety to reduce to a minimum any hazard to health in all groups of consumers" (FAO/WHO, 1958a).

The approach taken by the WHO/FAO Joint Expert Committee on Food Additives (JECFA) is that food additives should be allocated an acceptable daily intake (ADI) expressed as milligrams per kilogram body weight per day. This is not a toxic threshold, but is the quantity of an additive which may be consumed on a daily basis over a lifetime with no adverse effect.

The calculation of an ADI is based on the assumption that animal data can be extrapolated to man and that:

> some margin of safety is desirable to allow for any species difference in susceptibility, the numerical differences between the test animals and the human population exposed to the hazard, the greater variety of complicating disease processes in the human population, the difficulty of estimating human intake and the possibility of synergistic action among food additives (FAO/WHO, 1958b).

The ADI of an additive is typically calculated from the highest dosage of the substance which caused no effect in animal studies multiplied by a safety factor which takes into account the variability in response between humans and animals (usually a factor of ten) and the variability within the human species (usually a factor of ten). Therefore, typically the no observed effect level from the most sensitive species studied is divided by 100 (10×10) to yield the ADI. Biochemical variation and dynamics play a key role in arriving at the safety factor used in any given situation.

The safety assesment of additives which are to be consumed in large amounts—in the case of low-calorie foods, bulking agents and fat substitutes—presents special problems. For example, the difference between the amount that can be fed to an experimental animal and the amount normally consumed by man is small making the establishment of a no observable effect level difficult. In addition, impurities contained in the additive assume greater importance because of their relatively higher consumption. The criteria used in the safety assesment of these additives differ from those used to assess additives consumed in small amounts, such as high-intensity sweeteners. Greater emphasis is placed on their impurity profile and their effect on the nutritional content of the diet and also their influence on the bioavailability of nutrients in the diet. The 100 fold safety factor is inappropriate in calculating an ADI for these compounds and a lower one may be applied, particularly where the additive is similar to traditional foods, is metabolized into normal body constituents or displays a lack of overt toxicity.

In cases where an additive is found to be of extremely low toxicity it may be that no ADI need be specified. In this instance, the principle of *quantum satis* applies and the additive should be used within the strictures of good manufacturing practice (GMP). That is, it should be used at the minimum concentration required to achieve its technological purpose and it should not lead to adulteration of food of inferior quality nor should it create a nutritional imbalance

2.3.4   Estimating exposure

In order that the ADI set might have relevance to the consumer of the additive it is necessary to estimate the amount of exposure the population will have to any particular additive.

There are several methods for estimating this exposure. For example, JECFA (FAO/WHO 1967) favour the dietary survey approach which involves calculating the average daily intake of an additive based on: (a) levels arising from good technological practice; (b) average consumption of foods containing the additive; and (c) average body weight.

The *per capita* approach involves taking the total of the amount of an additive used in a country and dividing it by the total population of that country or comparing the total consumption of a particular foodstuff in a country with the normal level of additive used in that foodstuff.

Another method of assessing exposure is by market basket surveys which look at a 'typical' diet of a country and estimate the amount of a particular additive used in that diet. This approach does not take into consideration the small percentage of the population who are high users of products containing that additive.

2.3.5   Legislative control of additives

National governments are responsible for regulating food additives in such a way that consumption arising from natural occurrence added to consumption arising from deliberate addition to food does not exceed the ADI for each additive that is permitted. The WHO scientific group on procedures for investigating intentional and unintentional food additives have stated:

> it is desirable that national government should maintain a check on the total intake of each food additive, based on national dietary surveys, to determine whether the total load approaches the acceptable daily intake (WHO, 1967).

The simplest form of food legislation takes the 'negative list' approach. This attempts to prevent the criminal adulteration of food by forbidding the use of certain substances in certain foodstuffs. In principal, therefore, under a negative list system those substances not on the list are authorized. The EC Flavouring Directive (88/388/EEC) is an example of current legislation which has a negative list of substances which may not intentionally be added as such to foodstuffs or flavouring, although they may be present either naturally or following the addition of flavouring prepared from natural raw materials.

With the increased use of additives and the vast improvement in techniques for detecting and quantifying their use in foods, it has become necessary, and practical from the point of view of enforcement, to introduce a 'positive list' system. Here only additives which have been approved may be used and the levels at which they may be used are controlled.

Proposed EC legislation on additives consists of positive lists of approved substances. 'Conditions of use' tables limit the concentrations of additives which may be used in any particular category of food so that the amount consumed by a 'normal' person eating a 'normal' diet will not exceed the ADI for that additive. In drafting these conditions of use tables various factors are taken into consideration including the ADI of the additive, consumption studies and information provided by the food industry on the technologically desirable levels for the additives in food.

The EC legislation on additives is known as 'horizontal' legislation. This deals with foodstuffs on a general basis and covers such areas as labelling and packaging materials. 'Vertical' legislation deals with standards for specific products, for example jams, chocolate and honey.

At times vertical and horizontal legislation may appear to contradict each other. For example, aspartame is approved in the draft EC sweetener directive for use in energy reduced jams (horizontal legislation), yet it does not appear in the list of approved ingredients in the Council Directive on fruit jams (79/693/EEC) (vertical legislation). However, it seems likely that in instances such as these horizontal legislation will take precedence over vertical legislation.

United States legislation contains both negative and positive lists of additives. For example, amongst sweeteners, cyclamate is specifically banned from use in food whereas aspartame is approved for use in specified categories of food. No numerical limit is set on the amount of aspartame which may be used, the regulations stating that it may be used in accordance with good manufacturing practice. In practice this means the quantity of the substance added does not exceed the amount reasonably required to accomplish its intended physical, nutritive and other technical effect in food. GRAS substances, prior sanctioned food ingredients and food additives permitted in food on an interim basis (for example saccharin) are also included in individual positive lists. GRAS substances may have restrictions on their conditions of use and limits. For example thaumatin (a high intensity sweetener derived from *Thaumatococcus danielli*) may only be used as a flavouring adjuvant in chewing gum. In the case of saccharin, numerical limits on its use are set depending on the category of food it is approved for use in.

2.3.6   Format of a food additive application

The information required by the various regulating authorities for assessing the safety of an additive is supplied, by the manufacturer or sponsor of the additive, in the form of a food additive petition (FAP). A food additive petition is generally made up of the following elements:

1. The name, chemical composition and chemical identity of the additive.
2. Statement of the proposed use of the additive.
3. The intended technical effect of the additive.
4. A method of analysis for the additive in food.
5. Full reports of all safety investigations with respect to the additive.

In addition some authorities have requirements for data on the environmental impact of the additive (e.g. USA), or have a requirement to prove that there is a reasonable technological need for the additive and the purpose cannot be achieved by other means which are economically and technologically practicable (e.g. EC) (89/107/EEC).

More detailed guidelines on the requirements for the safety investigation of food additives have been drawn up by various bodies including the Organization for Economic Co-operation and Development (OECD, 1981), the Commission of the European Community (CEC) (67/548/EEC) and JECFA (WHO, 1987) and the USA FDA (FDA, 1982).

2.4 Controls on the composition of low-calorie foods

As mentioned in the introduction to this chapter, one of the purposes of legislation aimed directly at low-calorie foods is to ensure the nutritional integrity of these products. For example the EC has recently drafted a directive (EC, 1991) which will control foods intended for energy reduced diets.

Foods intended for energy restricted diets are defined in this draft directive as "specially formulated foods which when used as instructed by the manufacturer, replace whole or part of the total daily diet."

The draft goes on to define the uses to which low-calorie foods are put in order to ensure that a satisfactory balance of nutrients is retained in these products in spite of the reduction in calories. Three categories are defined:

- products presented as a replacement for the whole of the daily diet;
- products presented as a replacement for one or more meals of the daily diet;
- products presented as an important source of nutrients for use by persons following a restricted energy diet composed of selected common foodstuffs.

Also defined in the draft directive is the essential composition of foods for weight control diets in terms of energy, protein, lipids, dietary fibre, vitamins and minerals.

2.5 Novel foods

Increasingly, low-calorie foods are using ingredients such as fat substitutes which may be produced by novel manufacturing techniques including biotechnology. Legislation is being drafted in the EC (Com(92) final–SYN426) and the UK (DHSS, 1991) to control 'novel foods' which are defined in the UK as "foods or food ingredients which have not hitherto been used for human consumption to a significant degree . . . and/or which have been produced by extensively modified or entirely new food production processes." It seems likely that many new ingredients which may be developed in the future for use in low-calorie foods and do not fall under the definition of food additives will be classified as novel foods.

In the UK the assessment of novel foods is currently voluntary on the part of the manufacturer who must decide whether its new product falls within the definition of a novel foods. The level of the safety assessment required for a novel food then varies depending on how 'novel' it is. The amount of information required for a genetically modified organism is much greater than that required for a fat substitute which is an exisiting raw material with a novel use. For example, a genetically modified tomato requires an extensive dossier including a toxicological assesment, whereas a product such as the fat substitute Simplesse, which is made from an existing raw material put to a novel use, requires only nutritional studies.

The EC will shortly be putting similar requirements into European legislation in the form of a Council Regulation (Com(92) final–SYN426). It is proposed that a twin track system will be introduced whereby foods which have the greatest potential for impacting on food safety will be assessed centrally by the SCF and other novel foods will be assessed by national experts appointed by the member states.

The FDA have taken a different stance, specifically on foods derived from biotechnology. The FDA do not propose additional regulations and believe that control "should depend on the food's characteristic, not on the method by which it was derived" (FDA, 1992) The onus of ensuring the safety of a product will remain on the producer. If the transferred genetic material or the product of its expression are not generally recognized as safe then it will be regulated as if they were additives under Section 402(a)(1) of the Federal Food Drug and Cosmetic Act. This interpretation of the act also applies to 'novel foods' not produced by biotechnology such as the fat substitute Simplesse, which in the US was awarded GRAS status as an additive.

2.6   Labelling of low-calorie foods

The labelling of foods in general is in a state of flux at the moment both in the USA and in the EC. In the USA the 1990 Nutritional Labeling and Education Act is in the process of being implemented by the FDA with wide reaching consequences for the labelling of foods. In the EC various subsidiary directives and amendments to Council Directive 76/112/EEC relating to the labelling, presentation and advertising of foodstuffs are in the process of being adopted. In general the FDA requirements and rules on the labelling of foodstuffs are considerably more specific and elaborate than the Community's.

The control of labelling of foods in general has a threefold purpose.

- To prevent false or misleading claims
- To provide the consumer with nutritional information
- To provide medical information to special patient groups

2.6.1 Claims

Various descriptors are used by companies to identify their products to the consumer as a low-calorie food, e.g. reduced energy, lite, light, free from sugar, etc. The regulatory trend is to define these descriptors in order to protect the consumer from misleading claims.

In the United States proposed labelling regulations (FDA, 1993a) prohibit the use of any nutrition claim for a food unless it uses terms defined by FDA regulations. For example 'low calorie' is defined as no more than 40 calories per serving and no more than 40 calories per 100 g of food. The proposed definition of calorie-free is less than five calorie for each serving. The term 'lite' or 'light' implies a reduction of one third in calories as does the claim 'reduced'. If more than half the calories are from fat, that fat content must be reduced by at least 50% with a minimum reduction of at least 3 g fat in each serving. However, a 50% reduction in fat need not be accompanied by a one third reduction in calories to justify the lite/light descriptor. A low-fat claim will be allowed if the product has 3 g of fat in each serving and in each 100 g.

The required reduction of one third to justify the claim 'lite/light' may present problems to manufacturers who are developing products which complement current thinking on reducing the intake of saturated fats. In many reduced-calorie products the main source of calories is fat, not sugar. Because of the energy density of fat (9 kcal g^{-1}) it is difficult to reduce the fat content of a product sufficiently to meet the one third requirement, even by using fat substitutes, without affecting the taste and texture. In addition, it can be seen that difficulty will arise with these proposals when it comes to defining what the product claiming an energy reduction is being compared against.

The proposals speak of 'reference foods'. However, how can a standard fruit cake be defined? What is a normal ice cream? The FDA have tentatively suggested that as well as the manufacturer's own full calorie food, comparison can be made against a competitor's product.

In the EC, a draft directive is currently being circulated which will control claims concerning foodstuffs (EC, 1992). In comparison with the US rules, the proposed EC rules are considerably less exhaustive but potentially equally controversial. For example, the term 'light/lite' will be restricted to products with a reduced energy content only. This proposal is still far from being agreed on and it is unlikely that it will actually be adopted in its present form.

The delay in producing EC legislation controlling claims concerning foodstuffs has prompted the United Kingdom to come forward with its own proposals in the hope of influencing a speeding up of the EC process. The proposed amendments to its Food Labelling Regulations 1984 (MAFF, 1992) (which already have controls on slimming claims), will introduce further legislative controls on certain nutrition claims as recommended by the Food

Advisory Committee (FAC). These controls will cover claims for 'low fat/saturates/sugar/salt', 'no added sugar/salt', 'high fibre', 'more/less' of any of these nutrients and 'free from fat/saturates/sugar/salt'. Comparative claims will require at least a 25% reduction by comparison with a 'normal' product.

2.6.2 *Nutritional information*

Nutrition labelling of foods is controlled in the EC by the nutrition labelling directive (90/496/EEC). Under this directive nutrition labelling is optional unless a nutrition claim is made. This contrasts with the FDA's proposals on labelling (FDA, 1993b) which would make nutrition labelling obligatory on virtually all processed foods. However, in May 1989 the EC adopted a horizontal directive on the labelling and marketing of food for particular nutritional uses (PARNUTS) (89/398/EEC). Included in the vertical directives in the process of being drafted to supplement this Directive is a draft Directive on Foods for Energy Restricted Diets (EC, 1991) which has specific nutritional labelling requirement for low-calorie foods as follows:

- The available energy per 100 g ml^{-1} and per specified quantity proposed for consumption must be stated.
- The amount of minerals and vitamins per 100 g ml^{-1}, expressed as a percentage of the recommended daily allowance (RDA) in the case of products meant for the replacement of the whole of the daily diet.

It also has requirements for instructions for the preparation of the product and where necessary a statement as to the importance of following those instructions as well as a laxation warning for those products containing more than 20 g a day of polyols.

In addition products designed to replace the whole of the daily diet should have the following labelling:

- a statement that the product contains an adequate amount of all essential nutrients for the day;
- a warning to maintain an adequate fluid intake and that the product should not be taken for more than three days without medical advice.

For products which replace one or more meals of the daily diet or which are presented as an important source of nutrients for someone on an energy restricted diet, a statement must be made that the product is only of use as part of a calorie-controlled diet and that other foodstuffs will be a necessary part of the diet.

In the USA any food which purports to be of use in reducing or maintaining caloric intake or body weight is considered to be a food for special dietary use and is subject to restrictions in labelling (21 CFR 105.66). In addition, the terms 'substitute' or 'imitation' are used in connection with certain 'standardized' foods such as margarine, cheese and sour cream which may have high-calorie ingredients replaced by low-calorie ingredients or additives. In the latest American proposal on food labelling (FDA, 1993c) the terms substitute or imitation will no longer be obligatory. However, the nutritional requirements for such a product will be laid down. A 'substitute' food must be nutritionally equivalent to its standardized counterpart and must contain the ingredients used in the standardized food and, although calories or fat must be lowered, the food must contain the same amount of fat-soluble vitamins as the standardized food.

The proposed FDA regulations define serving and portion size for 139 specific food product categories (FDA, 1993d). Nutritional content on labels must refer to these standardized serving or portion sizes. The concept of portion sizes directly impacts on the labelling of calorie restricted ready made meals. The serving size of these products is necessarily smaller than a reference serving. It is proposed that the manufacturer of a calorie-controlled product would be permitted serving size values differing from those set by the FDA if they have filed with the FDA's CFSAN a summary of the weight control or weight maintenance plan and the specified serving size of the plan.

2.6.3 Medical information

Some components of low-calorie foods require special labelling which provides information about the possible effects of overconsumption of that component or advice to special patient groups concerning the use of that component.

At the moment in the United States all retail establishments which sell products containing saccharin must display prominently a notice to the effect that saccharin may be hazardous to your health as it has been determined to cause cancer in laboratory animals (21 CFR 101.11). Also in the United States, certain protein-containing products which are represented for use in dieting must carry a warning that without medical supervision the diet can result in death and the product should not be used by infants, children or pregnant or nursing mothers. For certain protein products containing more than 400 kcal per day a diet plan must be provided and the consumer instructed only to use that product in conjunction with the diet plan (21 CFR 101.17(d)).

Special consideration is given to diabetics in the labelling of low-calorie soft drinks in the USA. If a diet drink contains a blend of nutritive and non-nutritive sweeteners, the label must carry a statement that the product contains sugar and that it should not be used by diabetics without consulting their doctor. A similar statement must be carried on products containing sorbitol, mannitol and hexitol drawing the diabetics' attention to the carbohydrate content of that product. Products containing hexitols are further forbidden from using the claim 'sugar free' (21 CFR 100.130).

In Europe, the draft Sweeteners Directive (COM(92)255 final–SYN 423) requires that the labels of all products containing aspartame carry the advice that they 'contain a source of phenylalanine'. In many other countries this or similar wording is already used on a voluntary basis. The advice is aimed at people who have phenylketoneuria, a rare genetic disease characterized by an intolerance to phenylalanine. The draft sweetener directive will also make it obligatory to carry a warning that excessive use of polyols may induce a laxative effect.

2.7 Conclusion

The term 'low-calorie food' encompasses a whole spectrum of foods ranging from controlled-calorie prepared meals through ultra low-calorie protein dietary supplements to zero-calorie soft drinks. Therefore, for regulatory purposes, they cannot be treated as a discrete entity. The individual components of these products have different legislation depending on whether they are additives, novel foods or foodstuffs in the traditional sense of the word.

The purpose of these regulatory requirements is to maintain the integrity and wholesomeness of the food supply, to protect against fraud and to protect the consumers' health. Unfortunately for those who wish to sell a low-calorie product to a worldwide market, different countries and jurisdictions have chosen different ways of achieving this end. Thus the product contents and label must be tailored differently depending on the market in which it is to be sold. While the worldwide trend towards free trade and commerce is gaining momentum, it is clear that the marketing of low-calorie products will continue to be subject to diversant regulations for at least the next decade.

References

21 Code of Federal Regulations (CFR) §100.130. Office of the Federal Register National Archives Administration, US Government Printing Office, Washington, 1985.
21 Code of Federal Regulations (CFR) §101.11. Office of the Federal Register National Archives Administration, US Government Printing Office, Washington, 1985.
21 Code of Federal Regulations (CFR) §101.17(d). Office of the Federal Register National Archives Administration, US Government Printing Office, Washington, 1985.
21 Code of Federal Regulations (CFR) §105.66. Office of the Federal Register National Archives Administration, US Government Printing Office, Washington, 1985.
21 Code of Federal Regulations (CFR) §170.3(e). Office of the Federal Register National Archives Administration, US Government Printing Office, Washington, 1985.
21 Code of Federal Regulations (CFR) §409(c)(3). Office of the Federal Register National Archives Administration, US Government Printing Office, Washington, 1985.
COM(92) final–SYN 426. Proposal for a Council Regulation on Novel Foods and Novel Food Ingredients. Commission of the European Communities, Brussels.
COM(92) 128 final–SYN 332. Amended proposal for a Council Directive on assistance to the Commision and cooperation by Member States in the Scientific examination of questions relating to food. OJ No. C 107, 28.4.92, p.6. Commission of the European Communities, Brussels.
COM(92) 255 final–SYN 423. Proposal for a Council Directive on sweeteners for use in foodstuffs. 17.6.92. Commission of the European Communities, Brussels.
DHSS (1991) Department of Health Guidelines on the Assessment of Novel Foods and Processes. HMSO 1991 Report on Health and Social Subjects No. 38.

EC (1991) Draft commission directive on foods intended for energy restricted diet (/u/C1L/04/ 04/00/111/3268/91–EN Rev)1. Commission of the European Communities, Brussels.

EC (1992) Draft proposal for a Council directive on the use of Claims concerning foodstuffs. SPA/62/ORIG–Fr/Rev2. 22 November 1992. Commission of the European Communities, Brussels.

67/548/EEC/ Annexe V of the 6th amendment of the Directive on the Approximation of Laws of Member States Relating to the Classification and Packaging of Dangerous Substances. Commission of the European Communities, Brussels.

76/112/EEC. Council Directive on the approximation of laws of the Member States relating to the labelling, presentation and advertising of foodstuffs. OJ No. L262, 27.07.76, p. 149. Commission of the European Communities, Brussels.

79/693/EEC. Council Directive of 24 July 1979 on the approximation of the laws of the Member States relating to fruit jams, jellies and marmalades and sweetened chestnut puree. Commission of the European Communities, Brussels.

88/388/EEC. Council Directive on the approximation of the laws of the Member States relating to flavourings for use in foodstuffs and to source materials for their production. OJ No. L184, 22.06.88, p. 61. Commission of the European Communities, Brussels.

89/107/EEC. EC Council Framework Directive on Food Additives. OJ No. L40, 11.2.89, Annex II, p. 33. Commission of the European Communities, Brussels.

89/398/EEC. Council Directive. OJ No. L186; 30.06.89. Commission of the European Communities, Brussels.

90/496/EEC. Council Directive of 24 September 1990 on nutrition labelling of foodstuffs. Commission of the European Communities, Brussels.

FAO/WHO (1958a) General principles governing the use of food additives. First report of the Joint FAO/WHO Expert Committee on Food Additives. (FAO Nutrition Meetings Report Series No. 15; WHO Technical Report Series No. 129, pp. 14–15.)

FAO/WHO (1958b) Procedures for the testing of intentional food additives to establish their safety for use. Second report of the joint FAO/WHO Expert Committee on Food Additives. (FAO Nutrition Meeting Report Series No. 17; WHO Technical Report Series No. 144, p. 17.)

FAO/WHO (1967) Specifications for the identity and purity of food additives and their toxicological evaluation; some emulsifiers and stabilizers and certain other substances. Tenth report of the Joint FAO/WHO Expert Committee on Food Additives. (FAO Nutrition Meetings Report Series No. 43; WHO Technical Report Series No. 373, pp. 23–24.)

Food Additives Association (FAA) (1981) Food Sanitation Law, Food Additives in Japan, edition for 1981, p.1. Japan Food Additives Association, Tokyo, Japan.

FDA (1982) Toxicological Principles for the Safety Assessment of Direct Food Additives and Color Additives used in Food. Bureau of Foods, US Food and Drug Administration, Washington DC.

FDA (1992) Statement of Policy: Foods Derived from New Plant Varieties. Federal Register 57 (104), 29.5.92.

FDA (1993a) Food Labelling: Nutrient Content Claims, General Principles, Petitions, Definitions of Terms, Definitions of Nutrient Content Claims for Fat and Cholesterol Content of Food. US Food and Drug Administration, Federal Register, 58(3), pp.2414–2416, 6.1.93.

FDA (1993b) Food Labelling: Mandatory Status of Nutrition Labelling and Nutrient Content Revision, Format for Nutrition Label (Title 21, Part 1 and 101). Federal Register, 58(3), 6/1/93

FDA (1993c) Food Standards: Requirements for Foods Named by Use of a Nutrient Content Claim and a Standardized Term (Title 21, Part 130). Federal Register, 58(3), 6.1.93.

FDA (1993d) Food Labelling: Service Sizes (Title 21, Part 101). Federal Register, 58(3), 6.1.93.

Federal Food, Drug and Cosmetic Act (FFDCA) 201 (s).

MAFF (1992) Draft Food Labelling (Amendment) (Nutrition Claims) Regulations 199–, Ministry of Agriculture Fisheries and Food, March 1992.

OECD (1981) OECD Guidelines for Testing of Chemicals. Organization for Economic Co-operation and Development, Paris 1981.

SLV FS 1991:7.The National Food Administration's Ordinance with Regulations on Food Additives, p.4, §3. Upsala, Sweden.

WHO (1967) Procedures for investigating intentional and unintentional food additives. Report of a WHO Scientific Group. World Health Organization, Geneva. WHO Technical Report Series No. 348, p.6.)

WHO (1987) Principles for the Safety Assessment of Food Additives and Contaminants in Food. Environmental Health Criteria 70. World Health Organization, Geneva, 1987.

3 Low-calorie bulk sweeteners: nutrition and metabolism

F.R.J. BORNET

3.1 Introduction

Today's consumers expect more and more pleasure from food. They want it to be lower in fat, sugar and calories and to be able to maintain or improve their health condition and well being. Additionally, they are still requiring the sensory qualities they have come to expect from it, such as flavour, mouthfeel, taste and colour. These must be taken into account in order to develop new healthy ingredients with any success. In the field of sucrose replacement, the use of high-intensity sweeteners to develop low-calorie beverages has been a success. However, sweeteners must be employed in conjunction with low-calorie bulk ingredients in order to produce new low-calorie food products.

In response to the market demand, industry has developed low-calorie bulk ingredients to replace sugar, the majority of which are legally permitted in food applications at present in Europe and the USA. Most of the low-calorie bulk ingredients are non-digestible sugars.

3.1.1 Sucrose

Sucrose is the standard bulk sweetener. Most food applications investigated were originally developed with sweetness and other functional properties of sucrose in mind (Knecht, 1990).

3.1.2 Sweetness and taste profile

Consumers have become so accustomed to the sweetness of sucrose that any substitute must match it exactly. Sweetness and taste profile (no aftertaste) in pure sucrose are almost perfect by definition.

Its solubility and viscosity in solution are very specific. In products containing water or solid products that dissolve in the mouth, the viscosity of the sucrose solution gives a particular mouthfeel, hence the term 'bulk' used when describing it. As the heat of solution of sucrose is only slightly negative ($- 2$ kcal g^{-1}), it has no cooling effect in the mouth.

3.1.3 Physicochemical properties and food applications

The osmotic pressure of sucrose as well as its ability to bind water and thus decrease its activity in food explain why sucrose has been extensively used as a food preservative allowing a reasonable shelf life (jams, confectionery).

Sucrose is a non-reducing sugar and it is stable in a heated, neutral solution of up to 100°C. In acid solutions, it is inverted or it breaks down into two monosaccharide components – glucose and fructose, which are both reducing sugars. The reducing sugars obtained from sucrose interact with amino acids (Maillard reactions). These reactions are the basis for the browning and aroma–flavour formation associated with heating food (cake, cookies, pudding, etc.).

The interaction between sucrose and fats is characteristic. It is the basis for confection of chocolate, ice cream and bakery products and it is ideal for most food applications.

The price of sucrose is low and stable. Possible dental caries are the only drawback in the absence of oral hygiene and fluoride prevention. It has been said that sucrose is not tolerated by diabetics and that it contributes to heart disease but this has been recently and publicly refuted (Glinsman et al., 1986). However, its calorific value (4 kcal g^{-1}) may appear too high.

3.1.4   Ideal low-calorie bulk sweeteners

In soft drinks and in dry mix beverages, water being the bulk agent, direct substitution of a high-intensity sweetener for sucrose is simple. In baked or cooked food (cake) however when sugar is replaced by a high-intensity sweetener the product is no longer the same. Moreover, this substitution increases the energy density and the lipid content of the new product. Obviously, sugar not only sweetens cooked food, but it also ensures the optimal volume. The sugar removed must be replaced by a bulking agent to compensate for the loss of volume, yet it should not have the same calorie content (see Figure 3.1).

Ideally, low-calorie bulk ingredients as a substitute for sucrose should have significantly fewer calories than sucrose, possess physical and chemical properties which precisely match those of sucrose, provide secondary health benefits (such as being non-cariogenic, useful for diabetics, and having fibre-like effects), confer no negative side effects and be completely safe at all levels of consumption.

Theoretically, a sugar with 0 kcal g^{-1} should either be excreted in the stool after reaching the large intestine without being fermented or be excreted in the urine after being absorbed via the small intestine. The main low-calorie bulk ingredients which have been developed so far are non-digestible sugars (i.e. sugar alcohols, fructo-oligosaccharides, polydextrose). Most of these are legally permitted in food applications at present in Europe and the USA.

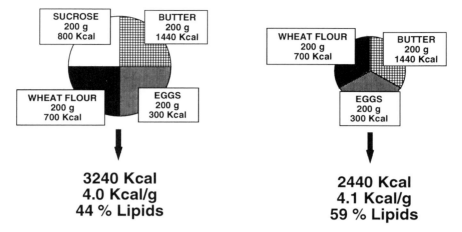

Figure 3.1 Nutritional imbalance for using high-intensive sweeteners without low-calorie bulk ingredient to develop low-calorie food.

3.2 Sugar alcohols

3.2.1 Sources and production pathways

Some sugar alcohols are present in fruits and vegetables but their extraction is scarcely a viable production pathway. They are industrially obtained under high temperature by catalytic hydrogenation of the relevant saccharides. Catalytic hydrogenation converts the aldehyde function of sugar into primary alcohol function and its ketonic function into secondary alcohol function. The hydrogenation linearises the chemical structure of sugars, improves chemical stability (absence of Maillard reaction) and modifies physicochemical and functional properties of sugars (higher affinity for water and lower capacity to crystallise). The hydrogenation of sugars dramatically reduces their bioavailability in the upper digestive tract and transforms them into non-digestible sugars.

Three categories of sugar alcohol chemical structures can be distinguished:

- Monosaccharides alcohols: sorbitol, mannitol, xylitol;
- Disaccharide alcohols: maltitol, lactitol, Palatinit®;
- Oligosaccharide alcohols: Maltidex®, Lycasin®.

3.2.2 Sorbitol

This natural sugar alcohol is present in many fruits, especially in the cherry and pear and in some fermented beverages such as cider (5–6 g l⁻¹). It is obtained industrially mainly by hydrogenation of glucose derived from starch (starch pathway; Figure 3.2) and from inverted sugar (sucrose pathway; Figure 3.3). It is available in both liquid and crystalline form.

3.2.3   Mannitol

This isomer of sorbitol is naturally present in the manna of the flowering ash, in figs, olives and algae. It can be produced by hydrogenation of mannose, a component of mannans and hemicellulose, but in industry it is produced by hydrogenation of fructose. Fructose can be obtained industrially by hydrolysis of sucrose (sucrose pathway) or by isomerisation of glucose (starch pathway). When fructose is hydrogenated, a 1:1 mixture of sorbitol and mannitol is obtained. Mannitol is much less soluble than sorbitol and it is removed by differential crystallisation.

3.2.4   Xylitol

In nature, xylitol occurs in fruit (raspberries), vegetable, mushrooms and algae. It is a pentitol sugar alcohol (a five carbon atom chain monosaccharide) obtained by hydrogenation of xylose. Xylose is industrially produced by hydrolysis of birch-wood xylans.

3.2.5   Erythritol

Erythritol is a tetritol sugar alcohol obtained by hydrogenation of erythrose. It is industrially produced through an aerobic fermentation of glucose

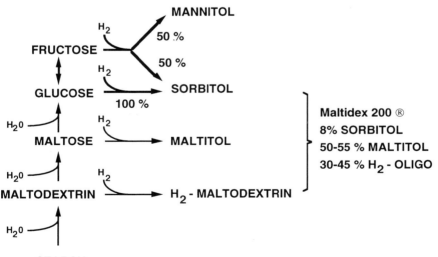

Figure 3.2 Scheme for industrial production of sugar alcohol from starch.

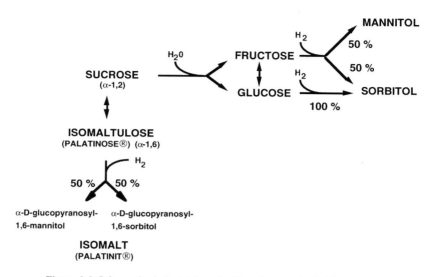

Figure 3.3 Scheme for industrial production of sugar-alcohol from sucrose.

by means of a yeast. It has a low molecular weight, a white crystalline aspect and is odourless.

3.2.6 *Lactitol*

Lactitol does not occur in nature. It is obtained by catalytic hydrogenation of lactose (Figure 3.4).

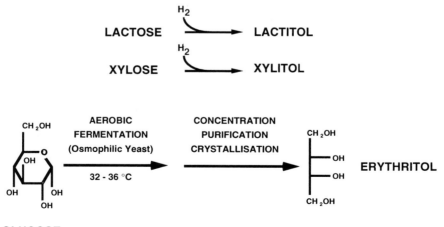

Figure 3.4 Principle of lactitol, xylitol and erythritol production.

3.2.7   Maltitol

Maltitol does not occur in nature. It is manufactured by the hydrogenation of maltose which in turn is produced by β-amylase hydrolysis of starch. Maltitol is available in both syrup and crystalline form. It is the main component of Maltidex® (Figure 3.2).

3.2.8   Isomalt (Palatinit®)

This disaccharide sugar alcohol is an equimolar mixture of two disaccharide alcohols (α-D-glucopyranosyl-α-(1→6)-sorbitol and α-D-glucopyranosyl-α-(1→6)-mannitol) obtained industrially by catalytic hydrogenation of isomaltulose (Palatinose; Figure 3.3). Isomaltulose is produced by catalytic isomerisation of sucrose by means of an enzyme system present in *Protaminobacter rubrum* bacteria. The α-(1→2) bond between glucose and fructose in the sucrose molecule is broken and linked in isomaltulose on α(1–6).

3.2.9   Hydrogenated glucose syrup

Hydrogenated glucose syrups are composed of a mixture in variable proportions of sorbitol (hydrogenated glucose), maltitol (hydrogenated maltose), maltotriol (hydrogenated maltotriose) and with hydrogenated tetra, penta and other high molecular weight maltodextrins (Figure 3.2). They are industrially produced from starch first by hydrolysis and then by hydrogenation of the glucose syrup. The hydrogenation acts on the terminal glucose unit of saccharide which is thus converted in sorbitol.

3.3   Physicochemical and functional properties of sugar alcohols

3.3.1   Taste profiles

The sweetening power of sugar alcohols is lower than that of sucrose. Their taste varies and their sweetness ranges from highest in xylitol to lowest in lactitol. Some sugar alcohols in the crystalline form are characterised by a pronounced negative heat of solution, producing an intense 'cooling effect'. Xylitol feels very cool because of its highly negative heat of solution (-153.07 kJ g^{-1}). Erythritol, which has a fairly negative heat of solution (-99 kJ g^{-1}), feels quite cool. Sorbitol and mannitol also produce a significant cooling effect, whereas maltitol and hydrogenated glucose syrup do not.

3.3.2   Solubility

Sorbitol and xylitol are very soluble in water whereas others, such as mannitol and isomalt are barely soluble. Maltitol and erythritol are fairly soluble. At 50°C the saturated solution of sorbitol contains 500 g l^{-1} water, twice that of sucrose (260 g l⁻¹). At the same temperature, only 45 g l⁻¹ mannitol are soluble. Hydrogenated glucose syrup cannot crystallise and acts as anti-crystallising agent in many food products.

3.3.3 Viscosity

The viscosity of sugar alcohol solutions depends on their molecular weight. The viscosity of hydrogenated glucose syrup is higher than that of sorbitol, maltitol or sucrose solutions.

3.3.4 Hygroscopicity

The hygroscopicity varies widely across the range of the sugar alcohols. Xylitol is very hygroscopic while mannitol, isomalt and erythritol have a very low hygroscopicity. Because of its low hygroscopicity, mannitol is mainly used as a dusting agent in confectionery tableting applications.

3.4   Fructo-oligosaccharides

3.4.1 Introduction

Fructo-oligosaccharides naturally occur in a large number of plants such as onion, asparagus, wheat, rye, triticale and Jerusalem artichoke (Clevenger *et al.*, 1988). These fructo-oligosaccharides are obtained industrially from sucrose or from inulin (fructan polymer) by an enzymatic process. ACTILIGHT® fructo-oligosaccharides result from the action on sucrose of a fructosyl furanosidase present in *Aspergillus niger*. Sucrose plays the dual role of fructose donor and fructose acceptor. The first reaction on two sucrose molecules, D-glucose (G) and D-fructose (F), results in kestose (GF2) and glucose. The same enzyme acts on kestose to produce nystose (GF3) and on nystose to produce fructosylnystose (GF4). Bonds between fructose units are β-(1–2). A chromatography processing step ensures the purification of fructo-oligosaccharides. The ACTILIGHT® composition is shown in Figure 3.5. The ACTILIGHT® range is available in both powder and syrup form.

3.4.2 Functional properties of fructo-oligosaccharides

Fructo-oligosaccharides of ACTILIGHT® have a taste profile similar to sucrose, without its cooling effect. When purified, the sweetness of fructo-oligosaccharides is 30% that of sucrose. Water retention capacity is higher than that of sucrose, similar to that of sorbitol. Being non-reducing sugars, fructo-oligosaccharides do not undergo Maillard reaction. They are

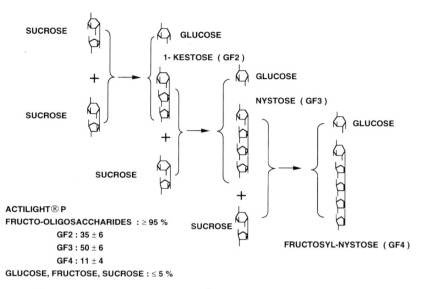

Figure 3.5 Principle of ACTILIGHT® fructo-oligosaccharides production.

not hydrolysed at pH values as low as 3 at temperatures up to 70°C and they are stable at medium pH at temperatures up to 140°C (Drevon and Bornet, 1992) (see Table 3.1).

Table 3.1 Functional properties of non-digestible sugars

Non-digestible sugar	Sweetness (Sucrose=1)	Taste of dry sugar	Stability		Viscosity	Hygroscopicity
			Heat(°C)	pH		
Sorbitol	0.70	Cool	< 160	2–10	Low	High
Xylitol	0.90	Very cool	< 160	2–10	Very Low	High
Mannitol	0.50	Cool	< 160	2–10	Low	Low
Erythritol	0.65	Cool	< 160	2–10	Very low	Low
Maltitol	0.75	None	< 160	2–10	High	Mild
Isomalt (Palatinit®)	0.60	None	< 160	2–10	High	Low
Lactitol	0.40	Slightly cool	< 160	2–10	Very Low	Mild
Maltidex®	0.75	None	< 160	2–10	High	Mild
Fructo-oligosaccharides (ACTILIGHT®)	0.30	= sucrose	< 140	> 3	= sucrose	Mild

3.5 Nutritional properties

3.5.1 Introduction

The main nutritional properties of non-digestible sugars and their interest with regard to human nutrition are related to their behaviour in the digestive tract and especially their capacity to reach the colon and to be fermented by microflora. The specific metabolism of these non-digestible sugars explains the digestive discomfort that can arise when ingesting them. Their digestible tolerance is widely influenced by the amount ingested, but it can be improved by other means.

3.5.2 Digestion–absorption

When sucrose is ingested, it is completely hydrolysed by brush border enzyme and absorbed in the small intestine. In subjects without urinary loss (i.e. without diabetes) all the glucose and fructose is metabolised by body cells and the calorific value of sucrose then reaches 4 kcal g^{-1}.

In the case of non-digestible sugars, a significant amount or all of the sugar ingested reaches the colon (see Figure 3.6). The consequences are multiple:

- significant loss of energy;
- production in gas (carbon dioxide, hydrogen, methane) which limits their digestive tolerance;
- reduction in the colonic pH via the short chain acid and the lactic acid production which modifies the status of the colonic microflora and its metabolism.

The monosaccharide alcohols (sorbitol, mannitol, xylitol) are slowly absorbed by facilitated diffusion. Compared to sucrose, their absorption is relatively low. Some disaccharide alcohols (lactitol) are non-digestible by brush border enzyme and reach the colon in totality (Patil et al., 1987). Maltitol and hydrogenated syrup are partially digested by α-amylase and maltase (Ziesenitz and Steber, 1987; Nilsson and Jayerstad, 1987; Baugerie et al., 1991). In vitro, the brush border enzymes are able to split the two constitutive saccharides of isomalt (Ziesenitz and Sieber, 1987). However the hydrolysis is lower than that of maltitol (Baugerie et al., 1989).

Erythritol has a different digestive fate because of its low molecular weight. Two recent studies (Hiele et al., 1993; Bornet et al., 1992) on ﾍealthy subjects have shown that after oral ingestion, erythritol is rapidly ﾍorbed by the small intestine and excreted unchanged in the urine. In ﾍ studies, 80% of ingested erythritol load was recovered in the urine ﾍ4 hours.

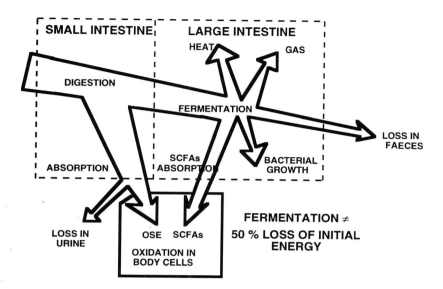

Figure 3.6 Fate of carbohydrate in the intestine.

There is no enzyme present in the small intestine which can specifically hydrolyse the (2–1)-β-glycosidic linkages found in fructo-oligosaccharides.

3.5.3   Digestive tolerance

The digestive tolerance of non-digestible sugars depends on the amount ingested, on the presence of factors reducing their osmotic load in the small intestine and on the degree of adaptation of the colonic microflora to perform fermentation.

The importance of the osmotic effect of non-digestible sugars is measured by the concentration of sugar leaving the stomach.

This obviously depends on the amount of non-digestible sugar ingested but also on factors reputed to slow down gastric emptying: calorie content of meal, solid content, viscosity, etc. The worst conditions in which to test the digestive tolerance of non-digestible sugars are encountered when fasting, when sugars are tested in a single liquid load and when the microflora of the subject has not been adapted by a chronic sugar ingestion. All these factors must therefore be taken into account in comparing digestive tolerance thresholds of different non-digestible sugars. The digestive tolerance of non-digestible sugars increases when sugars are ingested in a mixed meal, throughout the day or after a chronic exposure (see Table 3.2).

Table 3.2 Digestive tolerance doses of non-digestible sugars.

Non-digestible	Condition of testing			Dose	References
sugar	Single load	Throughout the day	Chronic exposure	(g)	
Sorbitol	+	–	–	10	Beaugerie et al. (1989);
	–	+	+	30–40	Jain et al. (1985); Rumessen and Gudman-Hoyer (1987); Van Es et al. (1986); Steinke et al. (1961); Pellier et al. (1990)
Maltitol	+	–	–	20	Beaugerie et al. (1989);
	–	+	+	60	Abraham et al. (1981)
Isomalt	+	–	–	20–30	Beaugerie et al. (1989);
(Palatinit®)	–	+	+	50	Thiebaud et al. (1984)
Lactitol	–	+	+	50	Beaugerie et al. (1989); Van Es et al. (1986)
Fructo-oligosaccharides (ACTILIGHT®)	–	+	+	30–40	Pellier et al. (1992)

3.5.4 Calorific value

Calorific value assessment of low-calorie bulk ingredients is being actively researched and it will be probably some time before any scientific consensus on a definitive method and on the standardisation of experimentation is reached. The calorific value of sugar alcohols has been recently reviewed (Bär, 1990; Bernier and Pascal, 1990; Voedingsraad, 1987). In humans the method that has been recently accepted by the Dutch and French authorities for nutrition labelling is the factorial method. It consists in measuring the amount of ingested sugar reaching the colon (using the terminal ilium incubation technique), and the amount of sugar recovered in the stool and the urine. The fraction absorbed in the small intestine and not excreted in urine provides 4 kcal after metabolism by body cells, while the fraction fermented in the large intestine has 2 kcal. The loss of energy when a sugar is fermented reaches approximately 50%. Part of it is due to the formation of short chain fatty acids and gas. The other part is due to the growth of bacteria which in turn release part of the energy as heat (Voedingsraad, 1987). The short chain fatty acids (acetate, propionate, butyrate) are rapidly absorbed by the colon and mainly used by the liver and peripheral tissues (muscle, adipose tissue) as energetic fuel.

Due to their digestive and metabolic behaviour, in theory non-digestible sugars have calorific value ranging from 0 to 3.2 kcal g^{-1}. The factor which has been previously described to modify the digestive tolerance by changing the orocaecal transit time may also modify the proportion of some polyols absorbed in the small intestine and thus their energetic value. The energetic value of some polyols rises when these are ingested in mixed meals or in the post-prandial period. It is therefore not easy to allocate a specific calorific value to each sugar alcohol for the purpose of food labelling regulations. Hence the application of an average calorific value for all polyols (2.4 kcal g^{-1}) adopted recently by the EC commission (90/496/EEC) (see Table 3.3).

3.5.5 Carbohydrate metabolism

Non-digestible sugars are not hyperglycaemic even when ingested alone. Sorbitol and xylitol which elicit low glycaemic and insulinaemic responses in healthy and diabetic subjects have been early proposed as a sucrose substitute in the diet for diabetes (Brunzell, 1978). Several studies have shown that maltitol elicits slow glycaemic and insulinaemic responses (Kearsley et al., 1982; Felber et al., 1987). Recently Debry and co-workers (personal communication) have shown that in the acute condition of ingestion, in healthy subjects, the glycaemic and the insulinaemic responses to 25 g maltitol in 250 ml water were significantly lower than the respective glucose and insulin responses to glucose and sucrose loads (see Figure 3.7).

Erythritol load (1 g kg^{-1} body weight in 2–5 l water) when taken in an acute oral tolerance test does not increase post-prandial plasma glucose and insulin levels in healthy subjects. Although nearly completely absorbed in the small intestine, erythritol is not metabolised and is excreted and recovered in urine (see Figure 3.8).

Table 3.3 Caloric value of non-digestible sugars (kcal g^{-1}) (adapted from Bernier and Pascal (1990) and Voedingsgraad (1987))

Non-digestible sugar	Condition of testing	
	Fasting	Post-prandial[*]
Sorbitol	2.0–2.6	3.3–3.9
Xylitol	2.0–2.6	3.3–3.9
Mannitol	1.5–1.9	?
Erythitol	0–0.4	?
Maltitol	2.8–3.2	3.5
Isomalt (Palatinit®)	2.4–2.9	?
Lactitol	?	1.4–2.5
Hydrogenated maltodextrins (Maltidex®)	2.8–3.2	3.5
Fructo-oligosaccharides (ACTILIGHT®)	2.0	2.0

[*]In mixed meal or out of a fasting period.

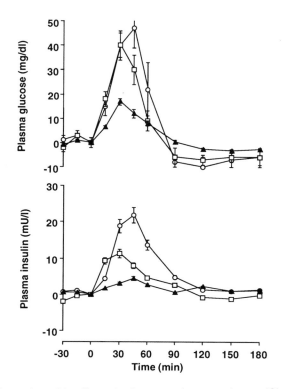

Figure 3.7 Glycaemic and insulinaemic plasma responses to glucose (○), sucrose (□) and maltitol (▲) ingestion (25 g in 250 ml water) in 8 healthy subjects (m ± SEM). (From Debry *et al.*, 1992, personal communication.)

The fact that no metabolism is taking place with erythritol has been recently confirmed in healthy human subjects by using a ^{13}C erythritol and $^{13}CO_2$ breath test method. After a 25 g ^{13}C erythritol single load, Hiele *et al.* (1993) have shown that no $^{13}CO_2$ breath excretion was detected during the 6 hours post-prandial period in any of the six healthy subjects tested. The same authors have shown that contrary to the other polyols, hydrogen in breath air does not rise after erythritol load because of its high small intestine absorption rate. This specific digestive behaviour of erythritol limits the risk of flatulence and diarrhoea (see Figure 3.9).

The fructo-oligosaccharides of ACTILIGHT® are not digested by the brush border enzyme of the small intestine (Oku *et al.*, 1984) and contrary to sucrose, 25 g fructo-oligosaccharides do not increase post-prandial plasma glucose or fructose levels. In diabetic subjects 8 g fructo-oligosaccharides per day for 14 days reduced the mean fasting

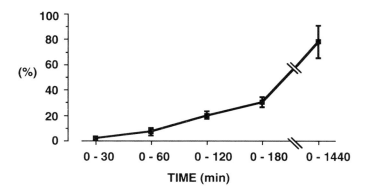

Figure 3.8 Kinetics of erythritol urine recovery over 24 h after oral erythritol (1 g kg⁻¹ body weight) ingestion in 6 healthy subjects (m ± SD). (From Bornet *et al.*, 1992.)

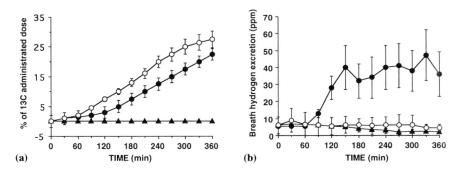

Figure 3.9 Cumulative amount of $^{13}CO_2$ excretion curves (in % of administrated dose) (a) and breath hydrogen excretion curves (b) after ingestion of glucose (○), lactitol (●) and erythritol (▲) (25 g in 250 ml water) in 6 healthy subjects. (m ± SEM). (From Hiele *et al.*, 1993.)

glucose levels (Yamashita *et al.*, 1984) (see Figure 3.10).

The improvement in glucose metabolism when using fructo-oligosaccharides could be mediated by the short chain fatty acid (SCFAs). Acetate and/or propionate given intravenously, orally or per rectal infusion were shown to reduce the serum free fatty acid concentration (Crouse *et al.*, 1968; Wolever *et al.*, 1989; Akanji and Hockaday, 1990) that inhibits glucose uptake. Acetate may be expected to worsen glucose tolerance by acting as a competitive substrate in the same way as free fatty acids. Recently Akanji and Hockaday (1990) have shown that this is not the case. Propionate has been shown to inhibit gluconeogen-

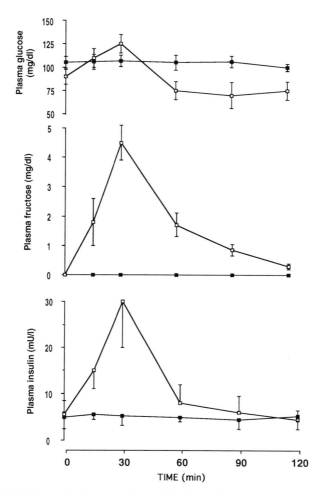

Figure 3.10 Glycaemic, fructosaemic and insulinaemic plasma responses to 25 g fructo-oligosaccharides (ACTILIGHT®) (■) or sucrose (□) ingestion in 6 healthy subjects (m ± SEM). (From Sano, 1986.)

esis and to stimulate glycolysis in isolated rat hepatocytes (Anderson and Bridges, 1984) with effects opposite to those of acetate. Long term oral propionate in healthy subjects (7.5 g sodium propionate per day for a period of 7 weeks) decreased fasting serum glucose and maximum insulin increment during glucose tolerance test (Venter *et al.*, 1990) suggesting that the improvement in glucose tolerance and insulin sensitivity may in part be mediated through the effects of propionate on hepatic carbohydrate metabolism.

3.6 Conclusions

Non-digestible sugars (polyols and fructo-oligosaccharides) are proposed as sugar substitutes because of their technological and nutritional properties. They are non-digestible or slowly digestible in the small intestine and when they reach the colon they are fermented by its microflora which reduces their calorific value. All non-digestible sugars elicit a slow glycaemic and insulinaemic response and may induce an improvement of insulin sensitivity via the liver and peripheral metabolisms of the SCFAs. In the colon, the fructo-oligosaccharides are specifically used by the colonic bifididobacteria. The reduction in intestinal pH in response to non-digestible sugars could be a protective factor against colon cancer. Further studies in humans would be necessary to specify the nutritional properties of such sugars.

References

Abraham, R.R., Davis, M., Yudkin, J. and Williams, R. (1981) Controlled clinical trial of a new non-calorigenic sweetening agent. *J. Human Nutr.*, **35**, 165–172.

Akanji, A.O. and Hockaday, T.D.R. (1990) Acetate tolerance and the kinetics of acetate utilisation in diabetic and non-diabetic subjects. *Am. J. Clin. Nutr.*, **51**, 112–118.

Anderson, J.W. and Bridges, S.R. (1984) Short-chain fatty acid fermentation products of plant fiber affect glucose metabolism of isolated rat hepatocytes (41958). *Proc. Soc. Exp. Biol. Med.*, **177**, 372–376.

Bär, A. (1990) Factorial calculation model for the estimation of the physiological caloric value of polyols. In: *Proceedings of the International Symposium on Caloric Evaluation of Carbohydrates* (ed. N. Hosoya) pp. 209–257.

Baugerie, L., Flourié, B., Franchisseur, C., Pellier, P., Dupas, H. and Rambaud, J.C. (1989) Absorption intestinale et tolérance clinique au sorbitol, maltitol, lactitol et isomalt. *Gastroentérol. Clin. Biol.*, **13**, 102 (A).

Baugerie, L., Flourié, B., Marteau, P., Pellier, P., Franchisseur C. and Rambaud, J-C. (1991) Digestion and absorption in the human intestine of three sugar alcohols. *Gastroenterology*, **99**, 717-723.

Bernier, J.J. and Pascal, G. (1990) Valeur énergétique des polyols (sucres alcools). *Méd. Nutr.*, **26**, 221–238.

Bornet, F., Dauchy, F., Chevalier, A. and Slama, G. (1992) Etude du devenier métabolique, après ingestion chez l'homme sain, d'un nouvel édulcorant de charge basse calorie: l'érythritol. *Gastroentérol. Clin. Biol.*, **16**, 169 (A).

Brunzell, J.D. (1978) Use of fructose, sorbitol, xylitol as a sweetener in diabetes mellitus. *Diabetes Care*, **1**, 223–230.

Clevenger, M.A., Turnbull, D., Inoue, H., Enomoto, M., Allen, J.A., Henderson, L.M. and Jones, E. (1988) Toxicological evaluation of neosugar: genotoxicity and chronic toxicity. *J. Am. College Toxicol.*, **5**, 643–662.

Council Directive on Nutrition Labelling (90/496/EEC).

Crouse, J.R., Gerson, C.D., Oscarli, L.M. and Liebers, C.S. (1968) Role of acetate in the reduction of plasma free fatty acids produced by ethanol in man. *J. Lipid Res.*, **9**, 509–513.

Drevon, T. and Bornet, F. (1992) Les fructo-oligosaccharides: ACTILIGHT®. In: *Le Sucre, les Sucres, les Édulcorants et les Glucides de Charges dans les IAA* (ed. J.L. Multon) TEC & DOC Lavoisier, Chapter 12, pp. 313–338.

Felber, J.P., Tappy, L., Vouillamoz, D., Randin, J.P. and Jequier, E. (1987) Comparative study of maltitol and sucrose by means of continuous indirect calorimetry. *J. Parent. Nutr.*, **11**, 250–254.

Glinsman, W.H., Irausquin, H. and Park, Y.K. (1986) Evaluation of health aspects of sugars contained in carbohydrate sweeteners. Report of sugars task force, 1986. *J. Nutr.*, **116** (11S); S1–S216.

Hiele, M., Ghoss, Y., Rutgeerts, P. and Vantrappen, G. (1993) Metabolism of erythritol in humans: Comparison with glucose and lactitol. *Br. J. Nutr.*, **69**, 169–176.

Jain, N.K., Rosenberg, D.B., Ulahannan, M.J., Glasser, M.J. and Pitchumoni, C.S. (1985) Sorbitol intolerance in adults. *Am. J. Gastroenterol.*, **80**, 678–681.

Kearsley, M.W., Birch, G.G. and Lian-Loh, R.H.P. (1982) The metabolic fate of hydrogenated glucose syrups. *Stärke*, **34**, 279–283.

Knecht, R.L. (1990) Properties of sugar. In: *Sugar—A User's Guide to Sucrose* (eds N.L. Pennington and C.W. Baker) Van Nostrand Reinhold, New York, Chapter IV, pp. 46–65.

Nilsson, U. and Jagerstad, M. (1987) Hydrolysis of lactitol, maltitol and Palatinit by human intestinal biopsies. *Br. J. Nutr.*, **58**, 199–206.

Oku, T., Tokunaga, T. and Hosoya, N. (1984) Non-digestibility of a new sweetener, 'Neosugar', in the rat. *J. Nutr.*, **114**, 1574–1581.

Patil, D.H., Grimble, G.K. and Silk, D.B.A. (1987) Lactitol, a new hydrogenated lactose derivative: intestinal absorption and laxative threshold in normal human subjects. *Br. J. Nutr.*, **57**, 195–199.

Pellier, P., Flourié, B., Franchisseur, C., Beaugerie, L., Dupas, H. and Rambaud, J.C. (1990) Tolérance clinique au sorbitol en situation de consommation habituelle, occasionelle ou régulière. *Gatroentérol. Clin. Biol.*, **14**, 87 (A).

Pellier, P., Flourié, B., Beaugerie, L., Franchisseur, C., Bornet, F. and Rambaud, J-C. (1992) Tolérance digestive à l'ingestion de bonbons contenant des fructo-oligosaccharides. *Gastroentérol. Clin. Biol.*, **16**, 181 (A).

Rumessen, J.J. and Gudman-Hoyer, E. (1987) Malabsorption of fructose-sorbitol mixtures. *Scand. J. Gastroenterol.*, **22**, 431–436.

Sano, T. (1986) Neosugar applications in diabetic patients. Presented at *Third Neosugar Research Conference*.

Steinke, J., Wood, F.C., Domenge, L., Marble, A. and Renold, A.E. (1961) Evaluation of sorbitol, in diet of diabetic children at camp. *Diabetes*, **10**, 218–227.

Thiebaud, D., Jacot, E., Schmitz, H., Spengler, M. and Felber, J.P. (1984) Comparative study of isomalt and sucrose by means of continuous indirect calorimetry. *Metabolism*, **33**, 808–813.

Van Es, A.J.H., De Groot, L. and Vogt, J.E. (1986) Energy balances of eight volunteers fed on diets supplemented with either lactitol or saccharose. *Br. J. Nutr.*, **56**, 545–554.

Venter, C.S., Vorster, H.H. and Cummings, J.H. (1990). Effects of dietary propionate on carbohydrate and lipid metabolism in healthy volunteers. *Am. J. Gastroenterol.*, **85**, 549–553.

Voedingsraad (1987). The energy value of sugar alcohols. *Recommendations of the Committee on Polyalcohols*. Netherland Nutrition Council, The Hague, June, 1987.

Wolever, T.M.S., Brighenti, F., Royali, D., Jenkins, A.L. and Jenkins, D.J.A. (1989) Effect of rectal infusion of short chain fatty acids in human subjects. *Am. J. Gastroenterol.*, **84**, 1027–1032.

Wolever, T.M.S., Spadafora, P. and Eshuis, H. (1991) Interaction between colonic acetate and propionate in humans. *Am. J. Clin. Nutr.*, **53**, 681–687.

Yamashita, K., Kawai, K. and Itakura, M. (1984). Effects of fructo-oligosaccharides on blood glucose and serum lipids in diabetic subjects. *Nutr. Res.*, **4**, 961–966.

Ziesenitz, S.C. and Sieber, G. (1987). The metabolism and utilisation of polyols and other sweeteners compared with sugar. In: *Development in Sweeteners*, (ed. T.H. Grenby). Elsevier Applied Science, London, Vol. 3, pp. 109–154.

4 Low-calorie bulking ingredients: nutrition and metabolism

G. ANNISON, C. BERTOCCHI and R. KHAN

4.1 Introduction

The low-calorie bulking ingredients are often identified as 'dietary fibre' which are generally recognised as the non-digestible components of food. Dietary fibres include cellulose, pectins, hemicelluloses, gums and mucilages, and lignins. They come from a variety of sources and are often chemically not well defined. This variability in quality and composition makes it difficult to describe their precise physico-chemical characteristics and hence it prevents their use in many food formulations. The ever growing need for good quality, low-calorie bulking ingredients to be used in low-calorie soft drinks, baked products, desserts and ice creams, has been recognised by the food industry.

For the purpose of this chapter a low-calorie bulking ingredient will be defined as a 'natural' or 'novel' food ingredient which provides foods and drinks with such organoleptic properties as body, texture, flavour, mouth-feel and taste. These attributes are found in non-digestible polymeric carbohydrates such as phycocolloids, cellulose, pectins, hemicelluloses and gums.

'Carbohydrates' is a general term used for a class of organic compounds which comprises monosaccharides (e.g. glucose and fructose), disaccharides (e.g. sucrose and maltose), oligosaccharides (e.g. cyclo-dextrin) and polysaccharides, (e.g. starch and cellulose). There are water-soluble and -insoluble carbohydrates, and some carbohydrates are digestible while others are not. The digestible polysaccharides (starch) are a major source of physiological energy. Carbohydrates like cellulose, pectin and hemicelluloses are classed as low-calorie bulking materials because they resist digestion in the small intestine. They may be partially or totally fermented in the large bowel by the gut microflora but, as will be discussed later, the energy contributions from these processes are low.

In this chapter, after a brief comment on the popularly known low-calorie bulking material, 'dietary fibre', the chemistry, physicochemical properties, digestion, metabolism in the body and the energy value of the individual non-digestible, low-calorie, soluble and insoluble polysaccharides in foods will be discussed.

4.2 Dietary fibres

4.2.1 Introduction

The term 'dietary fibre' lacks a clear definition and has been a subject of many interpretations. It was originally defined as plant polysaccharides with some lignins which are resistant to the hydrolysis by the digestive enzymes in man (Trowell *et al.*, 1985). The main components of dietary fibre are non-starch polysaccharides (NSP), but due to imprecise methods of analysis it also includes such minor components as oligosaccharides, polyphenolics (including lignin), cutin, waxes, suberin, phenolic esters and inorganic constituents. On the basis of the fact that these minor components differ considerably in their nutritive and physiological properties and that the levels of the individual components are difficult to analyse, it has been recommended that the term 'dietary fibre' should be obsolete and instead referred to as non-starch polysaccharides (NSP) (Anon, 1991).

4.2.2 Sources and functional properties

A 1987 survey (Anon, 1987) listed over 100 products or ingredients that include dietary fibre (NSP) available to the US food industry. The main sources for NSP are cereals, especially whole grain foods, vegetables, wheat, maize, rice, peas and sugar beet. The composition and the quality of NSP in these sources vary. For example, wheat, maize and rice contain mostly water-insoluble NSP, whereas in oats, barley and rye a significant proportion of NSP is water soluble. The main criteria that will affect both the dietary value and performance in food products is the ratio between soluble and insoluble NSP. The soluble NSP will influence the water absorption and its activity during the processing and storage of the food, such as bread, biscuits and extruded products. The particle size of NSP is also important because it will affect the ability to absorb water as well as influence the texture and mouthfeel. If the fibre ingredient is too coarse, it can produce a harsh or gritty texture. On the other hand, if it is too fine its water-holding ability may be reduced (Mongeau and Brassard, 1982). For most food formulations a bland flavour and neutral colour NSP is desirable.

Soybean fibres have been shown to contain a complex mixture of polysaccharides. The cellulosic component is mainly present in the soya hull fibres, whereas the cotyledon fibres are mostly composed of non-cellulosic polysaccharides, like arabinogalactans and acidic polysaccharides, such as pectins. Soybean fibres have been claimed to exhibit multiple physiological benefits, like the regulating effect on blood lipids, glucose metabolism and nutrients absorption. The sugar beet fibre contains on the average hemicelluloses (28%), pectins (25%), cellulose (24%), protein

(5%), ash (3%) and moisture (7%). The presence of both soluble and insoluble polysaccharides roughly in 2 : 1 ratio makes an interesting ingredient for cereal and baked products (Christensen, 1989).

4.2.3 Physiological effects

The low content of NSP in the diet of Western Society has been associated with such 'civilisation' diseases as constipation, obesity, cardiovascular diseases, diabetes, colon rectal cancer and others. Clinical research has indicated that NSP from different sources have different physiological effects. For example, cereals, with high contents of hemicelluloses, improve bowel activity, whereas NSP from fruits and vegetables, with a high proportion of pectin, have little or no colon activity, but a hypocholesterolemic action. These results have been confirmed using pure pectin and sugar (Stasse-Wolthuis, 1987).

Some adverse effects of NSP in elderly and growing children can be anticipated because of the anionic nature of some of the polysaccharides. For example, the uronic acid residues of pectins can complex and remove some of the essential divalent cations, such as calcium, iron, copper and zinc (Eastwood and Mitchell, 1976). However, *in vivo* studies in humans do not support significant reduction in mineral bioavailability except where phytate or oxalate is also high.

The report of the 'Panel on Dietary Reference Values of the Committee on Medical Aspects of Food Policy' recommends that adult diets in the UK should contain an average of 18 g per day of NSP from a variety of foods (Anon, 1991).

4.3 Low-calorie polysaccharides

4.3.1 Introduction

Polysaccharides are natural hydrophilic polymers of high molecular weight (Whistler and BeMiller, 1973). They may be branched or linear in structure. The physicochemical properties of polysaccharides are dependent on their structure. For example, in linear polymers like starch or cellulose, the straight chains can orient in parallel alignment so that a large number of hydroxyl groups along one chain are in close proximity to the hydroxyl groups of the other chain. In such a situation, the chains form an association through hydrogen bonding, resulting in aggregation of the chains and making the polymer insoluble in water. On the other hand, polysaccharides with irregular structure, due to branching, substituents and different types of monomeric residues, cannot align or associate so readily, and consequently they tend to be soluble in water, forming solutions that will not gel under normal conditions.

Polysaccharides are used in food formulations as a bland carrier for flavour and to provide appropriate viscosity, texture or mouthfeel, clarity and stability. These functions are achieved by exploiting the inherent properties of polysaccharides and their derivatives, such as gelatinisation and water-holding or thickening characteristics, gelling or non-gelling, binding or adhesive properties, film forming and emulsifying characteristics. Some of the important functional properties of polysaccharides relevant to food formulations are briefly described (Glass *et al.*, 1991).

4.3.1.1 Viscosity. The use of water-soluble polysaccharide to control solution and dispersion rheology is one of the most important functional features of polysaccharides. They modify rheology by virtue of their high molecular weights, chain entanglements and polymer–solvent interactions. Viscosity is the measure of the resistance of the flow of a liquid. More precisely, it is defined as the ratio of the shearing stress to the rate of shearing. Polysaccharides are particularly suitable for providing a high viscosity at a low concentration.

4.3.1.2 Gel-forming properties. Gelling behaviour of polysaccharides generally involves association of polymer chain segments at junction zones, whose formation usually requires a certain structural regularity of the polymers and favourable conditions for such chain associations. In the case of iota carrageenan, inter-chain associations occur primarily through double helixes (the junction zones) which can aggregate to form gel in the presence of certain cations. In the case of pectins, the network formation by junction zones is induced and stabilised by calcium ions which favour the formation of hydrogen bonds between the chains. This gelling property is obviously important in food processing (Pilnik and Rombouts, 1985).

4.3.1.3 Water-holding capability. Absorption of a large amount of water is typical of both soluble and insoluble polysaccharides. Soluble polysaccharides interact with water and affect the flow characteristics of the solution causing an increase in viscosity even at low concentrations. As the concentration increases, interactions with other molecules can occur, causing a further increase in viscosity. In some cases, the associations of polysaccharide chains result in the formation of a gel. In such cases a large volume of water is immobilised in an extended network of polysaccharide chains. Insoluble polysaccharides, which do not form gels, absorb a large volume of water into their hydrophilic matrix.

The water-binding capacity is important in food products where processing could affect the moisture content. For example, in processed meat, polysaccharides are used to keep the meat moist and tender.

4.3.1.4 Stabilisation of emulsions. Polysaccharides are used in low-calorie salad dressings to suspend flavourings and spices and to stabilise the emulsion. Polysaccharides such as alginate and xanthan gum are employed as emulsifying agents to stabilise many food products. Pectin is used to prevent casein flocculation in acid milk products. Guar gum is used in ice creams to prevent the growth of ice crystals.

4.3.2 Pectins

4.3.2.1 Introduction. Pectins are of great interest to many scientists and technologists because of their special chemical, biochemical and physical properties. A pectin can be classified as a polyelectrolyte, a complex polysaccharide, a low-calorie bulking agent, a ubiquitous source of nutrition and a gelling agent in foods (Fishman and Jen, 1986; Pilnik and Voragen, 1990).

4.3.2.2 Occurrence. Pectins are a class of polysaccharides found in the primary cell walls and intercellular layers in plants. They can be obtained from sources such as apples, citrus fruits, sunflower and sugar beet. The pectin content of apples and the rinds of citrus fruit on a dry weight basis are roughly 15 and 30%, respectively.

4.3.2.3 Structure (see Figure 4.1). At present, there is no universally agreed definition of pectins. The definitions given below are those which are used in commercial practice (BeMiller, 1986).

Pectic acids are galacturonoglycans with few or no methyl ester groups which may exhibit varying degrees of neutralisation. Salts of pectic acids are called pectates.

Pectinic acids are galacturonoglycans which have one or more methyl ester groups and which may exhibit various degrees of neutralisation. Salts of pectinic acid are called pectinates.

Pectins are complex galacturonoglycans but primarily polymers of

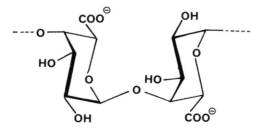

Figure 4.1 Structure of pectins.

D-galacturonic acid. The principal key feature of all pectins is a linear chain of (1→4)-linked α-D-galactopyranosyluronic acid units. It is often accompanied by neutral glycans, like arabinans, arabinogalactan and galactans (Khan *et al.*, 1983). White lupin seeds have been shown to contain (1–4)-linked β-D-galactopyranosyl residues in linear chains. Highly branched L-arabinofurans with no other monosaccharide residues have been obtained from mustard seeds.

Pectins are sub-divided according to their degree of methyl esterification. Pectins with greater than 50% degree of esterification are high-methoxyl pectins, and those with less than 50% are low-methoxyl pectins. Pectins from some sources (e.g. sunflower, sugar beet and potato) are known to contain acetyl ester groups which adversely affect the gelling properties of the pectin.

4.3.2.4   Physicochemical properties.   The solubility of pectin is determined by the degree of esterification, the distribution of the methyl ester groups, the pH, the molecular weight and the presence of counter ions in the solution. Monovalent cation salts of pectinic acid are usually soluble in water and di- and tri-valent cation salts are weakly soluble or insoluble.

Pectin solutions exhibit a non-Newtonian behaviour. The addition of monovalent cations to pectin solutions causes a reduction in viscosity, which is even more pronounced with decreasing methoxyl content (association). Soluble salts of di- and tri-valent cations show an opposite effect.

The most important property of pectin is its ability to form gels. The pectin chains interact over a portion of their length to form a network that entraps solvent and solute molecules. The size of these junction zones is critical in determining the nature of the gel. The gelation process is also dependent on the content of methyl residues and those of acetyl groups. The degree of gelation increases with the enhanced degree of methyl ester residues and decreases with the increased content of acetyl substituents. Other factors such as the pH, degree of amidation, heterogeneity and the presence of ions are also important.

4.3.2.5   Physiological properties.   Pectin has been shown to be a safe food ingredient for animal and for human consumption. It is degraded in the gastrointestinal tract but only slightly assimilated. The degradation is mainly caused by the microbial flora of the large intestine (*Lactobacillus*, *Enterococcus*, *Aerobacillus*, *Micrococcus*). The products of the breakdown do not appear to enter into the metabolism of the organism to an appreciable extent as pectin has been shown to provide a negative energy value.

Pectin has been reported to lower blood cholesterol levels and the low-density lipoprotein cholesterol fraction without changing levels of high-density lipoprotein cholesterol or glycerides. The decreased absorption of essential minerals has not been observed. Metabolic benefits have been claimed for the use of pectin in dietetic and diabetic foods (Behall and Reiser, 1986).

4.3.2.6 Food applications. Pectin imparts consistency and texture to the water phase of food products. It provides mouthfeel and spreadability to food but without calories. In a high-density energy drink sugar is normally used as a sweetener. In addition to its sweetness value it gives the drink mouthfeel and body. These latter qualities are lacking when a low-calorie soft drink is prepared using a high-intensity sweetener. Pectin can be used to achieve the required functionality in such applications.

4.3.3 β-Glucans

4.3.3.1 Source. Cereals, barley and oats are rich in β-glucans. The beneficial effects of dietary fibre, such as oat bran (7–8% of soluble β-glucan), has been previously discussed in the dietary fibre section.

4.3.3.2 Structure (see Figure 4.2). β-Glucans are glucose polymers containing both β-(1→3) as well as β-(1→4) linkages in various proportions depending on the source. The presence of β-(1→3) and β(1→4) linkages in the chain makes the polymer less linear and more water soluble than cellulose (Aspinall and Carpenter, 1984).

4.3.4 Galactomannans

4.3.4.1 Source. Galactomannans are found in the endosperms of some legume seeds (guar, tara and locust bean) where they are present as reserve polysaccharides. They are produced commercially from *Cyanopsis tetragonolobus* seeds and locust bean gum from carob seeds (*Ceratonia siliqua*) (Khan *et al.*, 1983; Stephen, 1983).

4.3.4.2 Structure (see Figure 4.3). In galactomannans the ratio of

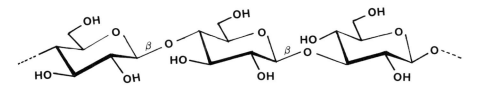

Figure 4.2 Structure of β-glucans.

mannose to galactose varies with its source. α-(1→6)-D-Galactopyranosyl units are distributed along a β-(1→4)-D-mannopyranoside chain, and are located on carbon-6. Treatment of galactomannans with an α-D-galactosidase and β-D-mannosidase indicates a block structure for the various galactomannans studied (Gidley *et al.*, 1991).

4.3.4.3 Physicochemical properties. Galactomannans with 18–24% galactose are insoluble in cold water but are soluble in hot water. Galactomannans with greater than 25% galactose are soluble in cold water to give highly viscous solutions. Viscosity of galactomannans is solely dependent on the nature of the backbone composed of D-mannose residues, provided that the D-galactose units present are sufficient to ensure solubility. In fact the β-(1→4)-mannan backbone of galactomannan is rather rigid and leads to high viscosities in dilute aqueous solution. Guar and locust bean gum polymers with different galactose contents show similar viscosity behaviour.

Galactomannans with low galactose content (less than 30%) form gel when used in combination with other polysaccharides (McClearly, 1979). Different degrees of interactions, with the same galactose content, with other polysaccharides such as kappa-carrageenan, agarose and xanthan have been observed.

4.3.4.4 Applications. Locust bean gum and guar gum are used in combination with carrageenan in low-calorie foods. When fat is removed from food products, the consistency and texture of the food is modified, spreadability decreases and the overall taste is altered. The mixture galactomannan and carrageenan has been shown to match the spreadability and sliceability of fat.

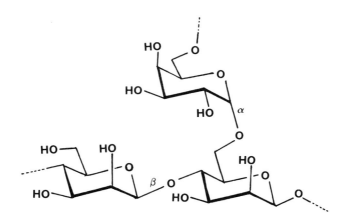

Figure 4.3 Structure of galactomannans.

4.3.5 Carrageenan

4.3.5.1 Source.   Carrageenan is a structural polysaccharide extracted from red algae (Rhodophyceae). Suitable species are collected in many locations or harvested from the sea by boat in the Far East and from the coasts on both sides of the Atlantic. In some locations seaweed farming is carried out by supporting growth on nylon threads (Painter, 1983a).

4.3.5.2 Structure (see Figure 4.4).   Various carrageenans have been isolated on the basis of their solubility in potassium chloride solution before and after treatment with alkali. There are six idealised carrageenans, namely iota, kappa, lambda, mu, nu and psi carrageenan. The kappa fraction is composed of D-galactose, 3, 6-anhydro-D-galactose and ester sulphate groups in approximate ratio of 5:6:7. The natural carrageenans, which are extracted from algal samples are mixtures of precursors, 'finished' molecules and molecules of an intermediate composition.

4.3.5.3 Physical properties.   Carrageenan is mostly soluble in water, although the solubility is influenced by several factors amongst which the most important is the chemical composition of the polysaccharide. Hydrophilicity of the molecule is determined by the number of sulphate groups present and the ratio of galactose to anhydrogalactose residues, the latter being highly hydrophobic. Solutions of carrageenan at concentrations below 3%, in the absence of ions that could promote gel formation, are highly viscous. At higher concentrations, formation of thermoreversible gels occurs in the presence of ions.

The strong negative charge retained over the normal pH range by carrageenan is the reason for its strong reactivity with positively charged polyelectrolytes. The strong interaction with proteins is a characteristic useful in many industrial processes. A special type of protein reactivity is exemplified by complexation of milk proteins by carrageenan. Non-gelling lambda carrageenan is used in products where thickening and stabilisation of cold milk is required, whereas kappa types find use in pasteurised products, being effective only after heating.

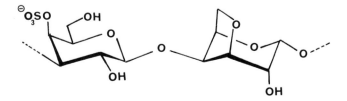

Figure 4.4 Structure of ϰ-carrageenan.

4.3.5.4 Applications.   Carrageenan is commercially used as a food ingredient in many products including dairy products, bakery products, meat products and water gels.

4.3.5.5 Physiological properties.   Carrageenan has been recognised as a natural low-calorie food additive. Rats fed on a carrageenan diet excrete the polysaccharide quantitatively in the faeces.

The sulphated polysaccharide showed some antipeptic activity, and with increased sulphate contents they exhibit anticoagulant activity.

4.3.6 Agar

4.3.6.1 Isolation and structure (see Figure 4.5).   Agar is a complex water-soluble polysaccharide which occurs as a structural carbohydrate in the cell wall of some algae. It is extracted from certain marine algae of the class Rhodophyceae. One type of agar is produced from the *Gelidium* species and another one from the *Gracilaria* species (Painter, 1983a; Indergaard and Ostgaard, 1991).

Agarose is considered to consist of chains having alternating (1→3)- and (1→4)-linkages with three extremes of structure: neutral agarose which contains (1→3)-linked β-D-galactopyranosyl and (1→4)-linked 3,6-anhydro-α-L-galactopyranosyl units; a 4,6-pyruvic acid acetal with small amounts of sulphate; and non-gelling galactansulphate with no or few 3,6-anhydro-L-galactopyranosyl and 4,6-pyruvated D-galactopyranosyl residues.

4.3.6.2 Physical properties.   Agar is insoluble in cold water but soluble in boiling water. It forms firm gels at very low concentrations. A 1.5% by weight solution, when cooled forms a firm resilient gel between 32 and 39°C, which does not melt below 85°C. The fact that gelation occurs at a temperature well below the gel melting temperature makes agar unique among the polysaccharides. Agar from different species exhibits different gelation temperatures, each of which is constant. The gelation temperature can be correlated with the methoxyl content of the gum. The melting

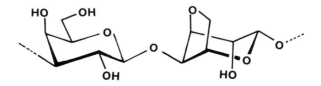

Figure 4.5 Structure of agar.

temperature of an agar gel is a function of concentration and of molecular weight.

Agar swells in water to give a solution with high viscosity at concentrations of 5 to 10%. The rheological behaviour is markedly influenced by the type of raw material and the extraction and purification processes used.

4.3.6.3 Applications.   In the food industry agar is predominantly used for its gelling, thickening and stabilising properties. The agar gel is resistant to heat which makes this hydrocolloid interesting for certain food applications. It has a unique ability for holding large amounts of moisture and provides bulk. It can therefore replace starch in breakfast cereals, non-starch bread and desserts.

4.3.6.4 Physiological properties.   Agar is an approved ingredient for food use and is on the GRAS list of the FDA. It is not metabolised by the human body. Because of its water-absorbing capacity it is used as a laxative.

4.3.7 Alginic acid

4.3.7.1 Source.   Alginic acid is a heteropolysaccharide extracted from brown algae, where it exists as the most abundant polysaccharide comprising up to 40% of the dry matter. It is located in the intercellular matrix as a gel containing various ions, such as sodium, calcium, magnesium, strontium and barium, which contribute to the strength and flexibility of the algal tissue. The world market value of algal polysaccharides is in excess of US $250 million per year (Indergaard and Ostgaard, 1991; Painter, 1983b).

4.3.7.2 Structure (see Figure 4.6).   Alginate is an unbranched binary copolymer of 1→4 linked β-D-mannuronic acid and α-L-guluronic acid of widely varying composition and sequential structure. The proportion and sequential arrangement of L-guluronic acid depends upon the kind of species of algae and the kind of algal tissue from which it is isolated.

4.3.7.3 Physical properties.   The sequential structure of alginate is crucially important for its functional properties. Viscosity is mainly dependent on molecular size, whereas the selectivity for binding cations is mainly related to the composition and sequence. This selective binding of cations to alginate accounts for the ability to form ionotropic gels. The blocks containing guluronic acid have high affinity to divalent cations such as calcium, strontium and barium, and it is the proportion of G-blocks in the polymer that determines the gel formation.

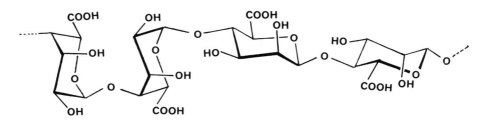

Figure 4.6 Structure of alginate.

4.3.7.4 Applications. Alginic acid exhibits such interesting properties as hygroscopicity, gelling, viscosity modifying and stabilising behaviour. For example, it can act as emulsifier and as emulsion stabiliser in low-calorie food where the fat content has been substantially reduced. In formulations where oils are required from zero to 50%, alginic acid with 0 to 0.5% can achieve the same functional properties.

4.3.8 Xanthan gum

4.3.8.1 Production. Xanthan gum is produced by *Xanthomonas campestris* cells grown in glucose as a carbon source. The microorganism is an efficient immobilised multi-enzyme system converting the carbohydrate substrate to the extent of 70% or more (Sutherland, 1989). The estimated world annual production of xanthans is in excess of 25 000 tonnes a year.

4.3.8.2 Structure. Xanthan gum is a branched extracellular polysaccharide with a glucopyranose backbone structure similar to cellulose and charged side chains with pyruvate and acetate groups. The quality of xanthan gum is dependent on the degree of substitution of the non-carbohydrate groups. Xanthans with varying amounts of acetates and pyruvates have been produced using other *Xanthomonas* species and different fermentation conditions.

4.3.8.3 Physical properties. The side chains of xanthan gums solubilise the normally insoluble cellulose backbone. Functional properties such as viscosity, gelling capacity, hydrophilicity and rheological behaviour are crucially important in the formulation of low-calorie foods. Xanthan gums are used for improving the rheological properties of low-calorie food products like dressings, frozen foods and fruit juices.

4.3.9 Polydextrose

4.3.9.1 Structure and synthesis. Polydextrose is a randomly linked, highly branched glucose polymer with a predominance of 1→6 bonds. It also contains a small amount of sorbitol as end groups and monoester bonds with citric acid. It is synthesised by thermal polymerisation of glucose in the presence of citric acid and sorbitol (Murray, 1988).

4.3.9.2 Physical properties. Polydextrose is highly soluble in water (up to 80%). Aqueous solutions of polydextrose behave as Newtonian liquids. Its solutions are slightly more viscous than sucrose solutions of the same concentration. It can be used in low-calorie soft drinks to provide the required viscosity and mouthfeel. These are stable for long periods of time at temperatures as high as 60°C.

Polydextrose is a good humectant and is effective in controlling humidity in food products. It retains moisture, avoiding large losses or gains of water in the food which could lead to prolonged shelf life and quality.

4.3.9.3 Applications. Polydextrose is a low-calorie bulking ingredient. Its properties such as humectancy, water-holding and viscosity modifying capabilities make it suitable for many food applications. It can replace the functional properties of sugar in several food formulations, except the sweetness. In some products it can also replace part of the fat. It has been claimed to improve the texture and palatability of low-calorie food products.

4.3.9.4 Physiological properties. Polydextrose is only partially metabolised by humans, it is poorly absorbed in the gastrointestinal tract and is not degraded by the intestinal flora. Only about 25% of polydextrose is metabolised which can be correlated to an energy value of 1 kcal g^{-1}. Polydextrose can be used in low-calorie food by replacing part of the sugar (energy value is about 4 kcal g^{-1} for carbohydrates) and fat (energy value is 9 kcal g^{-1}).

Polydextrose is approved for food use in the USA and many European countries.

4.3.10 Resistant starch

4.3.10.1 Structure. Starch consists of a mixture of varying proportions of two polysaccharides called amylose and amylopectin. Amylose is essentially a linear α-(1→4)-glucan with the occasional (1–2%) α-(1→6) linkage. Amylopectin is an α-(1→4) linked glucan with a higher proportion of a α-(1→6) linkages.

Table 4.1 Low-calorie bulking carbohydrates

Polysaccharide	Composition	Properties	Occurrence	Food applications
Pectin	$\alpha(1-4)$ D-Galacturonic acid Some ester groups	Gelling Thickening	Fruit Vegetable	Jams jellies Low-sugar or sugar free jams and jellies Beverages Milk products
D-Glucan	$\beta(1-4)$-D-Glucose ß-$(1-3)$-D-glucose	Bulking	Cereal (barley, oat)	Breakfast cereals
Galactomannan (guar gum, locust bean gum)	$\beta(1-4)$-D-Mannose backbone α-$(1-6)$-D-galactose	Thickening Stabilizing	*Cyanopsis tetragonolobus* (guar gum) *Ceratonia siliqua* (locust bean gum)	Sauces Salad dressing Ice cream Frozen foods
Carrageenan	Mixture of sulfated polysaccharides containing α-D-galactose and 3,6-anhydro-D-galactose	Thickening Gelling Protein reactivity	Rhodophyceae	Dairy products Bakery products Water gels Dessert gels Meat products Low-sugar jams Jellies
Agarose	β-D-Galactose and 3,6-anhydro-β-L-galactose linked-$(1-3)$	Gelling Stabilising Emulsifying	Rhodophyceae	Dairy products Confectionery Baked products Meat substitutes Dessert
Alginate	β-$(1-4)$-D-Mannuronic acid and α-$(1-4)$-L-guluronic acid	Water-holding Gelling Emulsion-stabilising Thickening	Phaeophyceae	Dairy products Bakery products Dietetic products Salad dressing Dessert puddings and gels Beer foam Stabilisation Fabricated foods
Xanthan gum	β-$(1-4)$-D-Glucose (backbone) D-Mannose D-Glucuronic acid	Thickening	*Xanthomonas campestris*	Beverages Canned foods Frozen foods Salad dressing Gels and puddings
Cellulose	β-$(1-4)$-D-Glucose	—	Widely distributed in plants	—
Polydextrose	D-Glucose	Thickening humectant	Synthetic products	Low-calorie soft drinks and food

4.3.10.2 Retrogradation. There is now evidence that a significant portion of the starch in some foods escapes digestion in the small intestine and enters the large bowel. Factors which affect starch breakdown by digestive enzymes include the degree of gelatinisation, the particle size, amylose content, interaction with other food components (NSP, protein and lipid), the presence of amylase inhibitors and the degree of retrogradation. Whilst it is inappropriate to discuss most of these factors in relation to low-calorie bulking agents it is possible that in the future retrograded starch will be utilised commercially as a bulking agent. Retrogradation is the process by which starch molecules (and in particular amylose molecules) associate closely together to form highly ordered structures (crystallites) which are resistant to α-amylase attack, hence the term resistant starch (Livesey *et al.*, 1990). Retrogradation of amylose can be promoted by the heating and cooling of solutions so that as much as 30% of the starch is retrograded (Gee *et al.*, 1991).

Retrograded starch can occur at low levels naturally in foods as a result of processing. Levels can be determined enzymatically, following dispersion of the sample in dimethylsulphoxide or strong base. This is a measure of chemically resistant starch. The starch which resists digestion in the small intestine is termed 'physiologically resistant starch'. Studies in ileostomates have demonstrated that starch other than retrograded starch can be resistant (Englyst and Cummings, 1990) to digestion in the small intestine. Thus *in vitro* resistance may not predict *in vivo* resistance and even when the *in vitro* method mimics closely physiological conditions, validation is still required by comparing the results with an *in vivo* model such as using ileostomates (Muir and O'Dea, 1992).

A summary of low-calorie bulking carbohydrates is given in Table 4.1.

4.4 Nutrition and metabolism

4.4.1 Introduction

Non-digestible polysaccharides are used as food ingredients in low-calorie products, because they resist digestion in the small intestine. They may be partially or totally fermented in the large bowel by the gut microflora but, as will be discussed later, the energy yields from these processes are low.

4.4.2 Digestion of polysaccharides in the foregut

Humans secrete a narrow range of enzymes capable of digesting polysaccharides. Essentially only α–(1→4) and α–(1→6)–glucan glycosidic linkages are digested by endogenous enzymes, which means that only starch and glycogen can be digested. Starch consists of a mixture of varying proportions of two polysaccharides called amylose and amylopectin. Amylose is essentially a linear α-(1→4)-glucan with the occasional (1–2%) α-(1→6) linkage. Amylopectin is an α-(1→4) linked glucan with a higher proportion of α-(1→6) linkages. Starch digestion begins with attack by α-amylases secreted in the saliva and from the pancreas. α-Amylases initially cleave starch with the formation of maltose, maltotriose and α-limit dextrins (α-(1→4), (1→6) oligosaccharide glucans). Further attack by the enzymes breaks down the maltotriose to maltose and glucose. These products are further degraded to glucose by the mucosal surface enzymes (sucrase–isomaltase complex, glucoamylase).

Modified starches which are finding greater use in the food industry are also resistant to attack by α-amylases and therefore escape digestion in the small intestine. In addition, some starch escapes digestion due to physico-chemical resistance. This 'resistant starch' will be discussed later.

All other polysaccharides described in the previous section, which are collectively termed 'non-starch polysaccharides' (NSP) are resistant to digestion by endogenous enzymes. The evidence that they pass through the small intestine unaffected has been based on the observations that no enzymic activity capable of degrading these polysaccharides has been detected in the intestinal content of humans, and that the ingested NSP is recovered quantitatively at the terminal ileum (Englyst and Cummings, 1985), although with some foods (potatoes, bananas) a small level of breakdown appears to occur in the small intestine (Cummings, 1988). Therefore in humans it can be predicted that polysaccharide-based low-calorie bulking agents will pass through the small intestine effectively unchanged. Interestingly, in the pig several studies have shown that considerable NSP digestion occurs prior to the large bowel which may be a result of the relatively much longer small intestine in the pig. This is almost certainly due to degradation by bacterial polysaccharides rather than by endogenous enzymes.

4.4.3 Degradation of polysaccharides in the large bowel

It is well established that carbohydrates, including polysaccharides, entering the large bowel are fermented to a lesser or greater extent by the microflora, and by-products, some of which can be absorbed, are used as an energy source (volatile fatty acids) by the host. The total energy available to the host is dependent on the extent to which a number of processes take place. For fermentation to occur the polysaccharides have to be broken down to their constituent sugars which are then absorbed by the microorganisms and fermented. Microorganisms break down polysac-charides by producing a large range of glycanases which cleave the glycosidic linkages of the NSP. Characterisation of glycanase activity in colon contents has not been extensive but studies of human faeces have shown that glycanases (lichenase, galacturonase, xylanase) and glycosidases (β-glucosidases, β-galactosidase, β-xylanase, α-fucosidase) are present and vary according to diet (Salyers, 1979). Studies by Bayliss and Houston (1985) demonstrated mannase, α-galactosidase and β-glucosidase activities in human faeces with the activity of the latter two being enhanced by the feeding of guar gum. Most of the activity was associated with bacterial cells. The feeding of a corn fibre residue (containing mainly cellulose and hemicellulose) to humans has also been reported to increase the levels of faecal β-glucosidase as well but β-glucuronidase activity was not affected. There is considerable difficulty in measuring the activity of these enzymes since isolates from gut often also contain substrate. The use of dyed polysaccharide substrates can overcome this problem and has been successful in demonstrating β-glucanase and β-xylanase activity in the gut contents of chickens (Annison, 1992).

The digestibility of polysaccharides varies considerably. In general, the more water-soluble the polysaccharide the more it is digested. However, it is probably only true for polysaccharides with structural features common to those which are eaten frequently in the diet. Polysaccharides from unusual sources or which are chemically modified may be resistant to glycanases elucidated by the gut microflora. The digestibility of polysaccharides also alters with time suggesting that the microbial population alters with changes in diet. The bacterial glycanase enzymes appear to be located on the surface of the bacterial cells which is also the location of the glycosidase enzymes which act on the oligosaccharides (Salyers, 1979). This allows the bacteria to utilise efficiently the monosaccharides as they are released but it is likely that for the complete breakdown of polysaccharides a cooperative effort by several species of bacteria is necessary (Cummings and MacFarlane, 1991).

4.4.4 Fermentation of carbohydrates

Monosaccharides entering the large bowel either as free sugars or as monomers of polysaccharides are taken up by bacteria and metabolised by the Embden–Meyerhof pathways to form pyruvate which then is converted to a number of products including short chain fatty acids (formate, acetate, propionate, butyrate), succinate, lactate, ethanol, CH_4, CO_2 and H_2 (Miller and Wolin, 1979). The fermentation is an anaerobic process providing four ATP molecules per hexose for the microorganism. Not all fermentation pathways provide the same products. The products are, however, surplus to the requirements of the bacteria and as will be discussed below, the volatile fatty acids (VFAs) may be absorbed and provide energy for the host. A theoretical yield of the products assuming that VFAs, methane and CO_2 are the sole products is that, 34.5 hexose molecules are converted to 48 acetate + 11 propionate + 5 butyrate + 23.75 CH_4 + 34.25 CO_2 + 10.5 H_2O. In practice, however, the ratio of the products may vary considerably depending on the nature of the substrate. Guar gum promotes propionate-rich fermentation whilst gum arabic enhances acetic and butyric acid fermentation (Telung *et al.*, 1987).

4.4.5   Metabolism of fermentation products

The gases produced from the fermentation of carbohydrates are mostly released as flatulence or are absorbed and subsequently lost from the body through the lungs. There is evidence that a portion of the methane is fixed in an acetogenic pathway by the hind gut microflora. In the ingestion of lactulose, pectin and resistant starch, methane and hydrogen production was less than predicted by stoichiometry (Christle *et al.*, 1992). A portion of the VFAs are absorbed and metabolised. Some metabolism may occur in the tissue of the caecum and the colon. Roediger (1980) has estimated that the cells of the colonic mucosa obtain 60–70% of their energy from bacterial fermentation products. Butyrate is a preferred substrate and is metabolised to CO_2 and ketone (Roediger, 1989). There is also evidence that butyrate is important for general lower bowel health with activities more widespread than simply acting as a fuel (Cummings and MacFarlane, 1991). Fatty acids which reach the venous portal system are transported to the liver. Propionate and butyrate are completely removed from the blood and metabolised by the liver but a portion of acetate escapes and enters the peripheral circulation. In the liver, propionate is a major precursor of glucose. Studies have suggested that propionate may have a role in cholesterol metabolism (Illman *et al.*, 1988), as dietary supplementation lowers serum cholesterol levels in rats either by inhibition of hepatic synthesis or by redistribution of cholesterol from plasma to the liver. In humans, however, no change in total cholesterol is seen when propionate is administered (Ventner *et al.*, 1990). Acetate is synthesised in the body as well as being absorbed from the colon following production through fermentation. The acetate is oxidised to provide energy in the peripheral tissues.

4.4.6   Energy value of non-nutritive bulking agents

Assuming 100% efficiency in digestion and absorption, the maximum amount of energy available from a particular food component, including carbohydrates, is equivalent to the gross energy (GE) value of the material. This can be determined experimentally using bomb calorimetry and is equivalent to the heat of combustion of the material. Different carbohydrates have different heats of combustion and whilst values for the mono- and oligo-saccharides are easily determined, the values for NSP are however not easily determined because of the difficulties in their isolation and purification. Livesey (1991a) has suggested that the GE of NSP can be estimated from the monosaccharide composition and has calculated values of 17.5, 16.8 and 16.5 kJ g^{-1} as averages for the NSP from cereals, fruit and vegetables, respectively.

In practice with many food components, digestion efficiency is less than 100% and energy is lost in faeces. The difference is termed digestible energy (DE). When energy losses occur in urine, the value obtained is the metabolisable energy (ME). A further value, net energy (NE), can be calculated to include energy lost through fermentation in the large bowel. In the case of ingested free glucose, absorption is highly efficient with negligible energy losses to the faeces, urine or to lower bowel fermentation. In this case GE, DE, ME and NE all have the same value (15.6 kJ g^{-1}). The energy values of free fructose and galactose are of a similar value since these sugars are highly digestible. The GE value of sucrose is 16.48 kJ g^{-1} and once again, due to the highly digestible nature of sucrose, the NE has the same value. Other highly digestible carbohydrates such as maltose and lactose (except in cases of lactose intolerance) will have similar energy values.

With other less well digested or metabolised carbohydrates such as the sugar alcohols, energy yields are less and the exact values are dependent on a number of factors including the extent of absorption, the amount excreted in the urine (either unchanged or as a metabolite), and the extent of fermentation of the material which reaches the large bowel. The metabolic fates of the sugar alcohols differ and it is clear that the energy yields from each will be different. Xylitol, being completely absorbed and metabolised, has a high energy value. In the case of erythritol, absorption is efficient (90%) and the material is subsequently excreted unchanged in the urine. The ME and NE values for erythritol are therefore very low (Tsuji *et al.*, 1990).

When most of the carbohydrate is not absorbed in the small intestine and moves into the large bowel the energy is made available through fermentation and the production of volatile fatty acids which are absorbed by the host. The total amount of energy available from the carbohydrate through fermentation can be estimated and is equivalent to about 12 kJ g^{-1}. This takes into account the loss of energy to the faeces in the form of bacterial cell mass which is about 0.3 kJ for each kilojoule of carbohydrate fermented (Livesey, 1991b). The net energy available from the fermentation is less than this due to other losses. The net energy from fermented carbohydrate can be predicted using the following relationship (Livesey, 1991b).

$$\text{Energy} = (1-A-B-C) \times D \times G \times H,$$

where the factors and their estimated values in parentheses are:

A = apparent efficiency in converting carbohydrate energy to faecal energy as bacteria (0.3)

B = efficiency of conversion to gaseous energy (0.05)

C = heat of fermentation (0.05)

D = proportion of carbohydrate fermented (variable)

G = gain of ATP per kJ for man for VFAs absorbed compared to gain from carbohydrate (e.g. for glucose = 0.85)

H = heat of combustion of carbohydrate.

This equation simplifies to 8.8 D. In the case where no fermentation occurs the energy value is 0 kJ and when fermentation is complete the value is 8.8 kJ g^{-1}. Lactitol is not absorbed in the small intestine but is completely fermented once it reaches the colon. Livesey (1990a) studied the NE value of isomalt, an equal mixture of glucosyl (α-1$\rightarrow$6) sorbitol and glucosyl (α-1$\rightarrow$6) mannitol in rats and pigs and reported its value also to be 8.4 kJ g^{-1}.

With the simple carbohydrates such as the sugar alcohols fermentation is essentially complete which accounts for the experimental values being so close to the theoretical values. In the case of polysaccharides (resistant starch and non-starch polysaccharides), which enter the large bowel the fermentation may frequently be incomplete. Livesey (1991c) reported that the digestibility across a range of dietary fibre components in a mixed Western diet was about 70%. The amount of energy available from carbohydrate (as volatile fatty acids) following fermentation is about 70% of the GE, thus the ME value of mixed dietary fibre components is approximately 50% (i.e. 0.7 × 0.7 = 0.49) or 8.4 kJ g^{-1}. Thus, in attempting to estimate the energy value of non-starch polysaccharide low-calorie bulking agents it is essential to have an estimate of the digestibility. With polysaccharides which are completely fermented (i.e. guar gum and gum arabic), the theoretical digestible energy value is 12 kJ g^{-1} (i.e. 17 × 0.7). The energy from polysaccharides which are essentially indigestible is theoretically 0.0 kJ g^{-1}. In practice the experimental values for polysaccharides are at variance with predicted values due the associative effects. It is now well established that the presence of polysaccharides in the diet can inhibit the digestion of other nutrients causing an increase in the energy content of faeces. The polysaccharides can also cause an increase in the excretion of endogenous material. In order to quantify this, the concept of partial digestible energy values has been introduced (Livesey, 1990b). Partial digestible energy and apparent digestible energy have the same value when there are no associative effects on other nutrients causing an increased loss of energy to the faeces. This is usually the case when sugar alcohols or oligosaccharides are considered (Livesey *et al.*, 1990).

Following studies in the rat, Davies *et al.* (1991) reported a partial digestible energy value of 10 kJ g^{-1} for guar gum. This is lower than the apparent digestible energy value (17 kJ g^{-1}) which can be calculated from its gross energy (17.5 kJ g^{-1}) and its apparent digestibility (98%). In the same study Davies *et al.* (1991) reported the partial digestible energy value of 0.0 kJ g^{-1} for Solka-floc (a purified cellulose), although an earlier study (Livesey *et al.*, 1990) indicated that this material was slightly digestible and had a partial digestible energy value of 0.8 kJ g^{-1}. Purified lignocellulosic materials from plant matter have recently been proposed as low-calorie flour substitutes in baked food products (Gould *et al.*, 1989).

Similar studies (Johnson, 1990) have been carried out on a commercially available (Beta-fibre®) mixture of sugar beet fibres (soluble and insoluble). The partial digestible energy was found to be 11.3 kJ g^{-1} with the non-starch polysaccharide component accounting for 9.1 kJ g^{-1}. The latter value is close to the expected value based on the digestibility and the efficiency of conversion of energy to bacterial cell mass. It suggests that the fibre product has little effect on the digestibility of other nutrients (Johnson, 1990).

Studies examining the energy value of resistant starches are few. Livesey *et al.* (1990) reported the partial digestible energy value of resistant maize starch and resistant pea (*Pisum sativum*) starch to be 15.0 and 12.4 kJ g^{-1} respectively. These values were lower than predicted from the apparent digestibility of starches data which was due to starches reducing the digestibility of protein. Such an effect has been observed with other 'fibre' but to a lesser extent.

Most of the studies described above have used the rat as a model. There is, however, evidence that the non-starch polysaccharides have similar effects on the digestion of other nutrients in human diets. Wisker *et al.*, (1988) reported that when six human subjects were fed a diet high in cereal dietary fibre there was a decrease in the digestibility of protein and fat and, by inference from dry matter digestibility, the starch. A more extensive study by Miles (1992) comparing the metabolisable energies of two diets (high fibre, low fat and low fibre, high fat) also demonstrated that the elevated levels of dietary fibre (from cereals, legumes, fruits and vegetables) decreased the digestibility of energy containing nutrients. The partial digestible energy value of the fibre was calculated to be 4.18 kJ g^{-1}.

Livesey (1990b) reported that the partial digestible energy of isolated dietary fibre components will be different from endogenous dietary fibre. The non-starch polysaccharides can effect the digestibility of other nutrients by entrapment. Such effects are less likely to occur with polysaccharide isolates, which means that these products are likely to have greater partial digestible energy values.

4.5   Conclusions

Non-starch polysaccharides are 'natural' products with reduced calories and therefore are used in low-calorie foods. The diversity in structure and functionality of natural polysaccharides offer scientists and technologists an opportunity to design and select bulk ingredients to suit their particular products. Mixtures of polysaccharides can also be used to achieve the desired organoleptic properties such as taste, viscosity, texture or mouth-feel, clarity and stability.

In order to exploit the full commercial potential of polysaccharides as low-calorie food ingredients their fundamental properties such as conformation, molecular weight and rheological behaviour must be understood.

References

Annison, G. (1992) Commercial enzyme supplementation of wheat-based diets raises ileal glycanase activities and improves apparent metabolisable energy, starch and pentosan digestibilities in broiler chickens. *Anim. Feed Sci. Tech.*, **38**, 105–121.

Anon (1987) *Cereal Foods World*, **32**, 556–565.

Anon (1991) In: *Dietary Reference Values for Food Energy and Nutrients for the United Kingdom*. RHSS 41, HMSO.

Aspinall, G.O. and Carpenter, R.C. (1984) Structural investigations on the non-starchy polysaccharides of oat bran. *Carbohydrate Polym.*, **4**, 271–282.

Bayliss, C.E. and Houston, A.P. (1985) The effect of guar gum on microbial activity in the human colon. *Food Microbiol.*, **2**, 53–62.

Behall, K. and Reiser, S. (1986) Effect of pectin on human metabolism. In: *Chemistry and Function of Pectins, ACS 310* (eds M.T. Fishman, and J.J. Jen). American Chemical Society, Washington, DC, pp. 248–265.

BeMiller, J.N. (1986) An introduction to pectins: structure and properties. In: *Chemistry and Function of Pectins, ACS 310* (eds. M.T. Fishman, and J.J. Jen). American Chemical Society, Washington, DC, pp. 2–12.

Christensen, E.H. (1989) Characteristics of sugarbeet fibre allow many food uses. *Cereal Foods World*, **34**, 541–543.

Christle, S.U., Murgatroyd, P.R., Gibson, G.R. and Cummings J.H. (1992) Production, excretion and metabolism of hydrogen in the large intestine. *Gastroenterology*, in press.

Cummings, J.H. (1988) Metabolism of dietary fibre in the large intestine. In: *The Role of Dietary Fibre in Enteral Nutrition* (ed. J.H. Cummings). Abbott International Ltd, Illinois.

Cummings, J.H. and MacFarlane, G.T. (1991) The control and consequences of bacterial fermentation in the human colon. *J. Appl. Bacteriol.*, **70**, 443–459.

Davies, I.R., Brown, J.C. and Livesey, G. (1991) Energy values and energy balance in rats fed on supplements of guar gum or cellulose. *Br. J. Nutr.*, **65**, 415–433.

Eastwood, M.A. and Mitchell, W.D. (1976) In: *Fibre in Human Nutrition*. Plenum Press, New York, p.109.

Englyst, H.N. and Cummings, J.H. (1985) Digestion of the polysaccharides of some cereal foods in the human small intestine. *Am. J. Clin. Nutr.*, **42**, 778–787.

Englyst, H.N. and Cummings, J.H. (1990) Non-starch polysaccharides (dietary fibre) and resistant starch. In: *New Developments in Dietary Fibre* (eds I. Furda and C.J. Brine). Plenum Press, New York.

Fishman, M.I. and Jen, J.J. (eds) (1986) *Chemistry and Function of Pectins, ACS 310*, American Chemical Society, Washington, DC.

Gee, J.M, Faulks, R.M. and Johnson, I.T. (1991) Physiological effects of retrograded α-amylase-resistant cornstarch in rats. *J. Nutr.*, **121**, 44–49.

Gidley, M.J., McArthur, A.J. and Underwood, D.R. (1991) ^{13}C-NMR characterization of molecular structure in powder, hydrates and gels of galactomannans and glucomannans. *Food Hydrocolloids*, **5**, 129–140.

Glass, J.E., Shulz, D.N. and Zubkoski, C.F. (1991) Polymers as rheology modifiers: an overview. In: *Polymers as Rheology Modifiers, ACS 462* (eds D.N. Schulz, and J.E. Glass). American Chemical Society, Washington.

Gould, J.M., Jasberg, B.K., Dexter, L.B., Hsu, J.T., Lewis, S.M. and Fahey, G.C. Jr. (1989) High-fiber, non-caloric flour substitute for backed foods. Properties of alkaline peroxide-treated lignocellulose. *Cereal Chem.*, **66**, 201–205.

Illman, R.J., Topping, E.L., McIntosh, G.J., Trimble, R.P., Storer, G.V., Talor, M.N. and Cheng, B.Q. (1988) Hypocholesterolaemic effects of dietary propionate studies. In whole animals and perfused rat liver. *Annals Nutr. Metabol.* **32**, 97–107.

Indergaard, M. and Ostgaard, K. (1991) Polysaccharides for food and pharmaceutical uses. In: *Seaweed Resources in Europe: Uses and Potential* (eds M.D. Guiry and G. Blunden) John Wiley & Sons, Chichester, pp. 169–183.

Johnson, I.T. (1990) The biological effects and digestible energy value of a sugar beet fibre preparation in the rat. *Br. J. Nutr.*, **64**, 197–199.

Khan, R., Wold, J.K. and Paulsen, B.S. (1983) In: *Rodd's Chemistry of Carbon Compounds* (ed. M.F. Ansell). Elsevier, Vol. I^{FG}, pp. 231–343.

Livesey, G. (1990a) Energy values of unavailable carbohydrate and diets: An inquiry and analysis. *Am. J. Clin. Nutr.*, **51**, 617–637.

Livesey, G. (1990b) The impact of the concentration and dose of Palatinit in foods and diets on its energy value. *Food Sci. Nutr.*, **42**, 223–229.

Livesey, G. (1991a) The energy value of carbohydrate and 'fibre' for man. *Proc. Austral. Nutr. Soc.*, **16**, 79–87.

Livesey, G. (1991b) Calculating the energy values of foods: Towards new empirical formulae based on diets with varied intakes of unavailable complex carbohydrates. *Europ. J. Clin. Nutr.*, **45**, 1–12.

Livesey, G. (1991c) Determinants of energy density with conventional foods and artificial feeds. *Proc. Nutr. Soc.*, **50**, 371–382.

Livesey, G., Davies, I.R., Brown, J.C., Faulks, R.M. and Southon, S. (1990) Energy balance and energy values of α-amylase (EC 3.2.1.1)-resistant maize and pea (*Pisum sativum*) starch in the rat. *Br. J. Nutr.*, **63**, 467–480.

McClearly, B. (1979) Enzymic hydrolysis, fine structure, and gelling interaction of legume-seed D-galacto-D-mannans. *Carbohydrate Res.*, **71**, 205–230.

Miles, C.W. (1992) The metabolisable energy of diets differing in dietary fat and fiber measured in humans. *J. Nutr.* **122**, 306–311.

Miller, T.L. and Wolin, M.J. (1979) Fermentations by saccharolytic intestinal bacteria. *Am. J. Clin. Nutr.*, **32**, 164–172.

Mongeau, R. and Brassard, R. (1982) *Cereal Chem.*, **59**, 413.

Muir, J. and O'Dea, K. (1992) Measurement of resistant starch: factors affecting the amount of starch escaping digestion *in vitro*. *Am. J. Clin. Nutr.*, **56**, 123–127.

Murray, P.R. (1988) Polydextrose. In: *Low-calorie Products* (eds G.G. Birch and M.G. Lindley). Elsevier Applied Science, London, pp. 83–100.

Painter, T.J. (1983a) Glycans of the Rhodophyta. In: *The Polysaccharides* (ed. G.O. Aspinall). Academic Press, New York, Vol. 2, pp. 207–233.

Painter, T.J. (1983b) Gycans of the Phaeophyta. In: *The Polysaccharides* (ed. G.O. Aspinall). Academic Press, New York, vol. 2, pp. 257–272.

Pilnik, W. and Rombouts, M. (1985) Polysaccharides and food processing. *Carbohydrate Res.*, **145**, 93–105.

Pilnik, W. and Voragen, A.G.J. (1990) Carbohydrates in food and feed. In: *Towards a Carbohydrate-based Chemistry*. Commission of the European Communities, pp. 43–76.

Roediger, W.E.W. (1980) Role of anaerobic bacteria in the metabolic welfare of the colonic mucosa of man. *Gut*, **21**, 793–798.

Roediger, W.E.W. (1989) Short chain fatty acids as metabolic regulators of ion absorption in the colon. *Act Veterinary Scandinavia*, Suppl. 86, 116–125.

Salyers, A.A. (1979) Energy sources of major intestinal fermentative anaerobes. *Am. J. Clin. Nutr.* **32**, 158–163.

Stasse-Wolthuis, M. (1987) Voedingsvezel. *Koolhydraten in Nederland*, **2**, 8–11.
Stephen, A.M. (1983) D-Mannans and D-galacto-D-mannan. In: Voedingsvezel. *The Polysaccharides* (ed. G.O. Aspinall) Academic Press, New York, Vol. 2, pp. 115–121.
Sutherland, I.W. (1989) Microbial polysaccharides, biotechnological products of current and future potential. In: *Biomedical and Biotechnological Advances in Industrial Polysaccharides* (eds V. Crescenzi, I.C.M., Dea, S. Paoletti, S.S. Stivala and I.W. Sutherland). Gordon and Breach Science Publishers, New York, pp. 123–132.
Telung, B., Remesy, C. and Demigne, C. (1987) Specific effects of guar gum or gum arabic on adaptation of cecal digestion to high fiber diets in the rat. *J. Nutr.*, **117**, 1556.
Trowell, H., Burkitt, D. and Heaton, K. (eds) (1985) *Dietary Fibre, Fibre-Depleted Foods and Disease*. Academic Press, London.
Tsuji, K., Osada, U., Shimada, N., Nishimurmura, R., Koboyshi, S., Ichikawa, T. and Hosoya, N. (1990) *Caloric Evaluation of Carbohydrates* (ed. N. Hosoya). Research Foundation for Sugar, Tokyo, p. 77.
Ventner, C.S., Vorster, H.H. and Cummings, J.H. (1990) Effects of dietary propionate on carbohydrate and lipid metabolism in man. *Am. J. Gastroenter.*, **85**, 549–552.
Wisker, E., Maltz, A. and Feldheim, W. (1988) Metabolisable energy of diets low or high in dietary fiber from cereals when eaten by humans. *J. Nutr.*, **118**, 945–952.
Whistler, R.L. and BeMiller, J.N. (eds) (1973) *Industrial Gums*. Academic Press, New York.

5 Fat replacer ingredients and the markets for fat-reduced foods

M.G. LINDLEY

5.1 Introduction

There is a growing perception that the food industry is increasingly driven by consumers rather than producers. The emphasis is shifting more and more from production to marketing. The days when producers tried to persuade consumers to eat what they were able to make are still with us to some extent, but seem gradually to be disappearing. As examples, few developments of the 'canned peas' or 'canned peaches' type can be expected in the future. In this environment, the consumer is setting the agenda for the food industry and the most successful companies are those that focus on satisfying the needs and wants of food consumers. They try to find out to what consumers aspire and then market products with attributes that will meet those aspirations.

However, consumer aspirations are usually merely expressed in general terms; the attributes being sought are quality, taste, convenience, nutrition, wholesomeness and value. Having defined their wants in this way, it then becomes the manufacturers' responsibility to interpret what these particular wants mean in terms of their own product range.

Increasingly, food companies are targeting products at particular market segments. Marketing to the masses is gradually being replaced by what is termed 'micromarketing'. This approach uses a variety of techniques to reach smaller groups of consumers that differ greatly in background, tastes and needs. The approach, characterised by an acknowledgement in the USA that "the mythological homogeneous America is gone", ultimately will lead to customised products aimed at smaller and more specific market niches. Already in the USA there is a shift away from mass advertising techniques to targeted promotions. Supermarket shelves now provide clear visible evidence of this increasing market fragmentation (Senauer *et al.*, 1991).

Despite this growing market segmentation, one unifying factor seeming to link almost all consumers is the belief that diet and health are inextricably linked. Western consumers generally, and American in particular, have embraced the 'healthy eating' crusade with great enthusiasm. Attempts to challenge Methuselah by a successful search for the 'magic bullet' are focused on healthier lifestyles, with diet being an increasingly important feature.

The contradictory behaviour of many consumers who may give up eggs, but eat super premium ice cream should not be permitted to deflect from the importance of these radical shifts in consumer behaviour. In the USA, such apparently conflicting habits are often called the 'workout–pigout' mentality, where the benefits of food that tastes good are balanced with the benefits of bodies that look and feel good.

Whether or not these contradictory habits affect (increase *or* decrease) longevity is, for the purposes of this discussion, irrelevant. What they provide is further illustration of the powerful influence that consumer lifestyles have on eating habits and hence food product developments and sales. Although the content of its message will almost certainly continue to change, the issue of diet and health will be with us for evermore. More importantly, consumers have found it simpler to absorb and react to 'negative' nutritional messages, best illustrated by the chronological trends of avoiding bread and potatoes, sugar, additives generally, and now fat and cholesterol. Thus, it should come as no surprise that attentions of the food industry are squarely directed at developing quality food and beverage products which respond to current 'fat and cholesterol' nutritional preoccupations.

The US Calorie Control Council conducted a survey in 1991 to examine trends in dieting and the use of low-calorie products. This survey showed that 141 million adult Americans consume low-calorie and/or reduced-fat foods and beverages on a regular basis (Table 5.1). Of these, two thirds are now consuming low or reduced-fat products. The consequences of these consumption patterns may also be exemplified by reference to the growth in new product introductions. Data from Gorman's New Product News (Table 5.2) clearly illustrate this dramatic growth, so much so that in 1990, 'reduced-fat' or 'reduced-calorie' claims were being made for approximately 10% of all new product introductions (McCormack, 1991).

These dramatic changes in consumer preferences send signals back to food manufacturers to develop innovations that meet demands for products with these characteristics. Thus, a multitude of fat replacer ingredients are being developed or have already been commercialised in direct

Table 5.1 Adult Americans consuming low-calorie/fat-reduced foods (source: Calorie Control Council 1991 national survey)

Category	Adult consumers (% population)
Use low-cal and low-fat	42.2
Use low-fat only	21.5
Use low-cal only	9.1
Non-users	24.2

Table 5.2 Light food and beverage product introductions (USA)

Year	Products introduced
1987	512
1988	475
1989	962
1990	1165

response to those consumer influences. These ingredients include wholly novel synthetic materials, proteins, carbohydrates and formulated products, all of which purport to restore to foods low in fat the sensory characteristics of their full fat equivalents.

The principal food sectors where lower fat foods have made market in-roads include margarine spreads, dairy desserts, baked goods, dressings and mayonnaises, cheeses and meat products. Recently, confectionery products have also been targeted.

This chapter will begin with a discussion of some of the key issues surrounding 'fat substitution', and the functionalities delivered to foods by fats and oils. Fat replacers from within each approach to fat replacement (synthetics, proteins, carbohydrates and formulations) will be selected on the basis of market importance, and described. Finally, some market data, both for fat replacers and for low- and reduced-fat foods will be presented.

5.2 Some issues surrounding fat substitution

5.2.1 Introduction

Fats and oils are important for their nutritional, functional and organoleptic properties. As the most concentrated source of energy, they supply approximately 9 kcal g^{-1}, over twice that delivered by proteins and carbohydrates. This explains why they are such targets for replacement by today's food industry.

Fats and oils are obtained from both animal and plant sources, those from plants being free of cholesterol. Fats from plant sources provide important essential fatty acid precursors for a group of hormones that regulate a variety of physiological functions. Fats and oils also act as carriers for essential fat-soluble vitamins. They aid the transfer of heat to food being fried and also contribute to a feeling of satiety after eating.

Fats and oils are important constituents of such diverse products as bakery goods, confectionery, dairy products, dressings and mayonnaises, margarines, salad and cooking oils.

Natural fats exhibit a wide range of physical properties which are influenced by the degree of unsaturation, the length of the carbon chain and the isomeric form of the fatty acids, the molecular configuration of the triglyceride and the polymorphic state of the fat. For example, fats consisting of highly saturated or long chain fatty acids will generally have a higher melting point than those possessing a high content of unsaturated or short chain fatty acids. Unsaturated fatty acids can have different configurations or isomeric forms which also have different melting points. They naturally exist in the *cis* form but can be converted to the *trans* form during partial hydrogenation. The type, quantity and distribution of fatty acids on the glycerol molecule also affect physical properties. Another important factor influencing functional performance is the crystalline state of the fat, due to the ability of fats to exhibit polymorphism, i.e. the ability to exist in more than one crystalline form.

Despite recommendations by health advisory organisations all over the world that people should decrease fat consumption, disappearance and sales data indicate that total fat consumption probably has not decreased significantly during the last 20 years. There has been a shift from saturated animal fats to polyunsaturated fats and oils, probably the result of educational efforts by health organisations and the influence of economic factors. For those individuals desiring to reduce their fat intake, the availability of engineered low-fat products might be helpful.

Current estimates indicate that the average North American consumer obtains 40% of his/her caloric intake from dietary fat. Recent figures from the UK National Food Survey published by the Ministry of Agriculture, Fisheries and Food indicate that in 1987 the percentage of food energy derived from fat was 42.2%; in 1988 it was 42.0% and during the first quarter of 1989 it was 41.8%.

With average fat consumption running at around 40% throughout the Western world, considerable impetus has been given to pronouncements from a whole range of health authorities as to what is the ideal percentage of energy intake derived from fat for the population as a whole. Although there is no precise consensus, it is generally recommended that the percentage of energy derived from fats and oils should be reduced to around 30% of total calorie intake. Some authorities also make recommendations on the proportions of saturated and polyunsaturated fats within that 30%, and also on the amount of cholesterol that should be consumed on a daily basis.

5.2.2 Disease risks

The driving force behind all of these well meaning recommendations on fat and oil consumption is the issue of health and nutrition. Coronary arterial diseases (atherosclerosis, thrombosis) and impaired cardiovascular circulation are major causes of morbidity and mortality in the West. In the USA there are estimated to be more than 500 000 deaths annually that can be put down to one form or another of coronary arterial disease. Other identifiable risk factors, i.e. smoking, elevated serum lipids, obesity, hypertension, inactivity and so on, may account for up to 50% of coronary arterial diseases.

In this regard, a strong association between plasma lipid levels, in particular low density lipoprotein, and coronary arterial disease (CAD) has been observed from both epidemiological data and clinical trials. Diabetes and obesity may also exacerbate the development of CAD. Knowledge of these risk factors and attention to their minimisation has been partially effective. The statistics from North America indicate that since 1964 there has been a 46% reduction in mortality from ischaemic heart disease and a 50% reduction in the incidence of strokes. These improvements partially reflect changing dietary habits (reduction in fat, both amounts and types) improved motivation in avoiding risk factors and more effective medical intervention, especially in treating high blood pressure.

Obesity is a major health problem. More than 30% of the population of the USA over 25 years of age is overweight. Although the aetiology is complex, excessive calorie consumption from fat and carbohydrates is involved in most cases. Obesity frequently predisposes the subject to hyperlipidaemia, hypercholesterolaemia, diabetes, hypertension and thus adversely affects health.

Diet plays an important role in cancer, the second major killer disease in the USA. There is a strong correlation between caloric intake, especially that from fat, and the incidence of many common cancers. Available evidence suggests that fat intake may be more relevant than total caloric intake. Dietary fat is a common factor in all these diseases and an enormous amount of research suggests that in general the contemporary Western diet provides excessive amounts of fat and cholesterol. As has been noted, on the basis of extensive clinical and epidemiological data there is a consensus that dietary fat intake should be reduced and that it should be reduced to match energy output and should not exceed 30% of calories. In addition, the fatty acid composition of dietary fat should meet certain guidelines.

In the UK, the Committee on Medical Aspects of Food Policy made a number of recommendations in 1984. Foremost among these was that the proportion of fat in the diet should be reduced so that the amount of energy derived from fats should fall from the 1984 level of 42% to a preferred 35% of the daily requirement. This requires a 17% reduction in the total fat intake. It has already been noted that current levels still refuse to come down from the 42% of energy derived from fats and oils. The Committee on Medical Aspects of Food Policy suggested that this reduction in energy intake from fats could be achieved in either of two ways; first, simply by reducing further the total amount of fat in the diet, or second, by altering the composition of the fat eaten so as to decrease preferentially the amount of saturated fats.

This overriding concern about the role of dietary fat in CAD, as illustrated by the pronouncement of the expert bodies, has tended to disregard the importance of lipids in determining food quality and the metabolic diversity of food lipids. This is due to the tendency to classify dietary fats solely as saturated or polyunsaturated and to judge fats simply on the basis of their effects on plasma lipids or lipoproteins. This has resulted in a negative image of food fats that overlooks many useful and crucial attributes.

The various components of food lipids perform many desirable organoleptic, physical, nutritional and biological functions that must be considered in making broad recommendations regarding dietary lipids. An understanding of these attributes and their mode of action should be helpful in developing more effective and perhaps safer strategies for motivating public acceptance of reduced-fat foods and in facilitating the fabrication of foods with less fat, but comparable satisfaction.

Fats and oils are important components in determining food selection. The organoleptic attributes of lipids in foods include contributions to aroma, flavour, colour, effects on texture, mouthfeel and overall sensory satisfaction and satiety. Edible fats and oils are excellent cooking media; they can be heated to above 100°C to provide rapid cooking and simultaneously impart surface texture and flavour to fried foods. Texture and consistency are important characteristics of edible fats and are determined by the relative concentrations of saturated and unsaturated fatty acids in the component triglycerides. The fatty acids have important functions in the application of edible oil. In this regard most of the fats used in contemporary vegetable oil, shortening and margarines have relatively high levels of unsaturated fatty acids for a specific consistency. This has been made possible by technical developments in hydrogenation and interesterification which represents major contributions from technology to provide an improved selection of dietary fatty acids and a range of functional ingredients for food formulation.

The food industry is caught in something of a dilemma. On the one hand nutritionists and consumer activists are pressing consumers to reduce the quantity of fats and oils in their diets. On the other hand, fats and oils are vital constituents of many food products, particularly if they are to be produced in a form that the consumer has become used to.

5.2.3   Nutrition and health

What is often not understood outside the scientific community is how important different lines of evidence are in arriving ultimately at a view concerning the aetiology and pathogenesis of a disease. This is nowhere more in evidence than in regard to coronary heart disease (American Heart Association, 1978). Evidence comes from animal and human studies, epidemiological studies of various kinds and clinical studies, studies which are uni-factoral or multi-factoral in design, and so on.

Furthermore, important as it is to resolve questions about the development of a particular disease, sight must not be lost of total mortality. It is quite clear that life expectancies are increasing in developed countries.

The roots through which food intake might operate ultimately on the heart are several and include the following:

- Obesity
- Serum lipids
- Blood pressure
- Platelet aggregation
- Coagulation
- Coronary vascular reactivity
- Cardiac membrane stability
- Cardiac substrate metabolism.

Although much attention is correctly focused on serum cholesterol as a particularly consequential pathway, other pathways should not be neglected. Moreover, some of the differences seen when a uni-factoral approach is taken to interpopulation studies may be attributable to differences in the ways in which these different pathways are operating.

Quantitative food factors which may influence coronary heart disease include the following:

- Energy balance
- Energy density
- Intake of dietary fibre
- Dietary fat
- Quality of fat
- Cholesterol intake
- Alcohol intake
- Intake of minerals.

Of particular value for hypothesis testing are the different trends in coronary heart disease mortality in different developed countries. In particular, rates have been falling for men in the United States of America, Australia, Canada, New Zealand, Belgium, Finland and Japan. In Sweden the rates are increasing, although from rather lower initial rates than in other developed countries, and in Eastern Europe rates are also increasing. There has been little change in coronary mortality rates in England and Wales.

Trends in coronary heart disease mortality are different for women than for men. The decline in coronary mortality in several developed countries started earlier and led to a greater divergence in life expectancy between men and women. It may be that dietary factors operate differently in women. Could it be that women have watched their saturated fat and therefore their polyunsaturated/saturated fat ratio for longer than men? If so, this may not have been due to concern about coronary heart disease, but for other reasons such as concern about obesity.

As has been noted, it is generally recommended that dietary fat intake should be reduced to match energy output and should not exceed 30% of calories (Haumann, 1986). In addition, the fatty acids composition of dietary fat should meet certain guidelines. Thus saturated fatty acids should not exceed 10% of calories and polyunsaturated fatty acids should not exceed 10% of calories. The remainder should be composed of monoenoic fatty acids. In addition, cholesterol intake should be 100 mg per 1000 kcal per day, sodium less than 3 g per day and dietary fibre around 25–30 g per day. While individual variability in susceptibility to risk factors should be recognised, adherence to these guidelines for food choices and lifestyle appears prudent in avoiding heart disease. The food industry can help this by providing food products with the appropriate fatty acid components.

These dietary recommendations have been developed for the chronic diseases that generally begin to appear in persons around 40 years old. There is some concern about the validity of these guidelines for the total population, especially for young, actively growing people. On the other hand, it has frequently been suggested that if such diets are not detrimental, their adoption should not be discouraged. In this context, it should be recognised that many of these degenerative diseases may have long development periods and be undetected by clinical tests. More definitive information is needed about the aetiology of these diseases and the capacity of dietary manipulation to delay their development.

In spite of recommendations and the trends in incidence of coronary arterial diseases, it is noteworthy that the average per capita consumption of fat is remaining remarkably constant in the UK.

Fat consumption levels are, however, decreasing slowly in the USA. There, the available data indicate the intake of fat is around 80–100 g per day providing 38% of calories. This is down from 41% of calories in 1977. Within this figure, saturated, monoenoic and polyunsaturated fatty acids supply 16, 15 and 7% of calories, respectively. Therefore, although total fat intake is being reduced, the consumption of saturated fatty acids should be reduced still further. Approximately 54 and 46% of dietary fat are obtained from animal and plant sources, respectively. Cholesterol consumption is derived from eggs (>50%), meats (approximately 30%) and dairy foods (15%).

In the context of diet and nutrition, food lipids serve as a source of energy, provide essential nutrients and assist the absorption of fat-soluble vitamins. Dietary lipids are hydrolysed by pancreatic lipase and the fatty acids and monoglycerides released are absorbed in the upper segment of the small intestine. Once absorbed, dietary lipids perform many diverse and vital metabolic, structural and regulatory functions.

The fat-soluble vitamins A and D function as bioactive signalling agents and in view of the strong pressure to reduce overall lipid intake, the potential impact on the intake and functions of fat-soluble vitamins must be considered. This applies particularly to those vitamins which are provided in significant amounts by foods of animal origin. The possibility that low-fat diets might result in marginal intakes of vitamins A and D, especially for the young and elderly, needs to be examined.

Overall, humans appear to possess remarkable adaptability and tolerance to wide ranges of intake of different fatty acids. Knowledge of the links between dietary fatty acids and the incidence and severity of degenerative diseases provides further rationale for modifying the lipid profiles of existing food products and developing new food products to improve nutrition and the quality of life of this and future generations. With these observations as background, the continuing drive for fat and oil substitutes which will assist consumers in meeting dietary guidelines and so improve their health prospects, has sound justification.

5.2.4 Consumer acceptance and labelling

Nutrition experts and marketing specialists expect calorie conscious consumers to accept fat substitutes with the same degree of enthusiasm they have displayed towards sugar substitutes. Financial analysts claim that the market potential may match or even surpass the success of intense sweeteners, particularly given the number of products that contain fat.

Although this is a somewhat simplistic view of the world, these observations do raise important issues that safety and regulatory authorities must address. Of particular concern is the control of the amounts of fat substitutes that may be consumed by the population at large. Since fat substitutes might be consumed by all sectors of the population, regulatory authorities must examine the safety of these materials with even more rigour than they traditionally show towards new materials for which approval is being sought. To exemplify, a new intense sweetener might make up substantially less than 1% of the food in which it is used; on the other hand, a fat substitute could theoretically represent up to 80% of some food items.

As a result, the safety testing of fat replacement ingredients may create scientific problems not normally encountered with other food additives. Really, the question boils down to one of how to test the safety of complete foods in a meaningful way. Normal safety testing of additives requires that test animals are dosed with sufficiently high levels of material to induce an effect. Through further tests, it becomes possible to explain the reasons for the effect, and also to define a 'no-effect level'. Acceptable daily intakes are then based on a fraction, usually 1/100th, of the no-effect level. Clearly, however, such an approach is not feasible for bulk ingredients such as fat substitutes. These factors help to explain why regulatory agencies have not felt able to reach a conclusion on fat substitutes such as sucrose polyester from Procter and Gamble.

In addition to the issues surrounding safety and the regulation of fat substitutes, there are labelling issues that also need to be addressed with foods so formulated. This is particularly relevant in the USA where the Food and Drug Administration (FDA) requires that a food be labelled as 'imitation' if it resembles another food and can be substituted for it, yet is nutritionally 'inferior' to the food it imitates. Logically, 'imitation' labelling should concern vitamin and protein contents more than fat content, but the wording of the laws currently requires that a reduction in calories would cause a food to be 'imitation'.

5.2.5 Technology

With fats and oils contributing such a broad range of functional attributes to finished food products it is difficult to see how a single means of substituting for fat in foods could possibly be successful. Consequently, a variety of ways in which oil-like properties can be conveyed to foods are being examined. These include the following:

- Non-caloric compounds having fat-like properties but whose ester bonds have been modified. Examples are sucrose polyester (Olestra) and polyglycerol ether (PGE).
- Non-caloric compounds whose structures differ significantly from those of triglycerides, such as polysiloxane.
- Structurally modified fats which are metabolised, but deliver fewer calories than normal fats. Examples are the carboxy/carboxylate esters from RJR-Nabisco and caprenin from a Procter and Gamble/ Grindsted joint venture.
- Hydrocolloids or proteins which bind large quantities of water as a gel or cream, exhibiting fatty-like mouthfeels while delivering approximately 10% of the calories of the fat they are claimed to be able to replace. Examples include modified starches from Avebe (Paselli SA2), A.E. Staley (Stellar), National Starch (N'Oil) and many others, gelled pectin from Hercules (Slendid) and microparticulated protein from NutraSweet (Simplesse).
- Formulated products which function in a similar way to the starches and proteins in that they bind large quantities of water, such as Avicel from FMC.

- Formulated products, e.g. Veri-Lo 100 from Pfizer, which contain some fat, but are blended with emulsifiers and other approved ingredients and designed to replace oil on a 1:1 basis.

Selected examples from within each of these categories are now discussed.

5.3 Fat substitutes and replacers

5.3.1 Introduction

It has been estimated that there are almost 200 products on the market or under development which purport to be able to substitute for some or all of the fat in selected food products. A comprehensive review of all these ingredients is impractical within a chapter such as this, and therefore selected examples will be discussed which illustrate the range of functional characteristics and diversity of products, and their applications.

5.3.2 Fat substitutes

5.3.2.1 Olestra. In the late 1960s, Procter and Gamble were working on the development of a new, easy-to-digest, high-calorie diet fat for premature babies and patients suffering from various disorders involving intolerance of natural fats and oils. They hoped to achieve this by esterifying fatty acids not with glycerol as in natural fats and oils, but with sucrose (table sugar), a disaccharide with eight hydroxyl groups. The first results were encouraging: the less complex esters (mono-, di-, and tri-esters) from sucrose and the fatty acids were found to have physical and (bio)chemical properties comparable to those of their natural counterparts. The tri-esters in particular proved to be an excellent substrate for lipase, the fat-splitting enzyme in the human gastrointestinal tract. However, a surprising discovery was made with the more complex esters: as the number of fatty acids linked to the sucrose moiety increased, the breakdown and uptake of the resulting ester in the intestine declined. For sucrose hexa-, hepta- and octa-esters, practically no breakdown or uptake could be observed. The densely packed tentacles of the octopus like molecule appear to cause so much steric hindrance that the lipase has too little room to manoeuvre close enough to the ester linkages.

Procter and Gamble realised that this fortunate finding was potentially far more promising than their initial aim. So the first fat substitute was born; research and development efforts began to develop and bring to commercial reality the mixture of sucrose hexa-, hepta- and octa-esters, under the collective name of sucrose polyester (SPE). Patents describing a sugar fatty acid ester or sugar alcohol ester with a least four acid ester groups, each fatty acid having from 8 to 22 carbon atoms, were first published in 1971.

Olestra is synthesised by a solvent-free reaction involving three principal steps:

(i) interesterification of sucrose with long chain fatty acids;
(ii) refining;
(iii) extraction.

It is probable that the production of Olestra is relatively expensive compared to the process of producing traditional vegetable oils which it will be targeted to replace.

The physical properties of Olestra depend on the fatty acids used in its preparation. For example, Olestra made from unsaturated fatty acids is a free flowing liquid. On the other hand, Olestra made from saturated or long chain fatty acids is a high melting solid at room temperature. Taste, appearance and functional characteristics are claimed to be indistinguishable from those of triglycerides containing the same fatty acids. Viscosity is claimed to be in the range of that of a typical vegetable oil at room temperature and to be higher than that of triglycerides with the same fatty acids. Procter and Gamble claim that Olestra is stable to repeated heating and cooling.

Olestra acts as an organic solvent in the intestine but has no caloric value as it is not broken down or absorbed. However, it is claimed that Olestra does not interfere with triglyceride hydrolysis and thus does not inhibit triglyceride absorption. It is also claimed, and there is substantial medical evidence for this, that Olestra increases cholesterol excretion. When some of this medical work was first published it probably led to Olestra being considered as having a drug-like action and hence may have contributed to some of the safety and regulatory difficulties Procter and Gamble appear to be having.

This will clearly be a considerable marketing hurdle to overcome should Olestra be approved and reach the market place. Another safety concern is the reported effect of Olestra on fat-soluble vitamins. Some studies have shown that vitamin E absorption was significantly lower in subjects consuming Olestra than those in a control group. As a result Procter and Gamble have obtained patents which recommend the use of vitamin fortified mixtures along with the consumption of Olestra. Again, this will present the company with a significant marketing hurdle to overcome.

Olestra has been proposed for use as a calorie-free replacement for fats and oils in quantities of up to 35% by weight in shortenings and salad and cooking oils intended for use in the home and food service industry. In commercial environments, it has been proposed as a 75% substitute for use in deep fat frying, especially for fried snack foods. Procter and Gamble petitioned the FDA for clearance of Olestra in shortenings, salad oils and salted snacks, while also publishing compositions for salad oil, prepared icing and cake mixes, mayonnaise, margarine and salad dressings. Olestra may also be employed in ice cream, peanut butter and processed cheese. Patents have also been published describing the use of Olestra in milk shake beverages, low-calorie baked products, stable emulsions in cake frosting bases, desserts, bread spreads and in emulsifiers. In other words, Olestra has the potential to be a completely versatile fat sustitute should it eventually reach the marketplace and should it be approved for the full range of applications for which it is claimed to be suitable. Therefore, Olestra has the potential to have a major impact on the development of reduced-calorie foods.

It is perhaps this versatility that will present Procter and Gamble (and FDA) with their final, possibly insurmountable, regulatory hurdle. Along with this versatility, of course, comes excessive potential exposure to consumers, and regulatory agencies may not be willing to approve the use of such a material for possible use in such a complete cross section of the food supply.

The development of Olestra has been a frustrating experience for Procter and Gamble for they have had to overcome many serious obstacles over the years. Summarising some of the more important issues Proctor and Gamble have been forced to tackle, mention must be made of the following:

1. Since Olestra is not broken down or taken up in the digestive tract, it arrives at the anal sphincter unchanged. The sphincter is designed to hold back something much more solid, and cannot contain the liquid SPE mass adequately. The result is 'anal leakage', a sort of diarrhoea. To address this problem, Procter and Gamble researchers then developed (and patented) other versions of Olestra with a melting range above 37°C by using fatty acids with longer chains and/or hydrogenated palm oil as a viscous additive. This approach does overcome the 'anal leakage' issue since Olestra then arrives at the anal sphincter as a solid fat, not a liquid as previously. Although one key issue is therefore solved, it must be remembered that a good synthetic 'fat' needs a melting range below 37°C to ensure it literally melts in the mouth. Also, by blending Olestra with palm oil, the 'zero calorie' platform cannot be used.

2. Fat-soluble substances such as cholesterol, triglycerides, lipoproteins and certain vitamins (A, D, K and, above all, E) dissolve easily in the SPE stream flowing through the digestive tract. A certain amount of the former is carried along with it to pass out of the body, instead of being taken up into the blood stream through the intestine. There- fore, it would appear that by reducing fat intake, the inevitable consequence of reduced vitamin uptake also occurs. Procter and

Gamble therefore patented a version of Olestra formulated with added vitamin E to guard against a deficiency of this particular vitamin. While this approach will work well when Olestra is not subjected to high heat regimes, it should be remembered that one of Olestra's primary intended uses is as a frying fat. This use would mean that any added vitamin E would decompose thermally. Vitamin deficiency therefore remains a possible issue of widespread use of Olestra, particularly as a frying fat.

3. Passive uptake of minute quantities of undigested Olestra in the intestine remains a regulatory concern. Clearly, it is difficult to prove a 'negative' such as this under all conceivable conditions.

4. Environmental questions may also remain, although whether these are 'real' or 'imagined' is unclear. Admittedly, research is necessary to establish whether there are microorganisms which can break down these types of substrates. If there is none, of course, the possible environmental problems are easy to contemplate.

5. Food legislation in the relevant countries is not necessarily designed to deal with an ingredient like Olestra. Although many countries have been happy to accept safety data on other bulk ingredients such as polydextrose and the sugar alcohols, the 'zero calorie' value of Olestra clearly makes difficult the design of appropriate long term tests.

Despite these well publicised difficulties being experienced by Procter and Gamble, the anticipated rewards for success have induced many other companies to enter this field. As a consequence, several companies are developing synthetic fats or chemically altered fats, but none has been approved, or is expected to be approved in the near future.

5.3.2.2 *Esterified propoxylated glycerol.*   Arco Chemical, a subsidiary of Atlantic Richfield, is working on chemically modified fats. Its esterified propoxylated glycerols (EPGs) are naturally occurring fats with propylene glycol inserted between the glycerol and fatty acid segments (Hamm, 1984).

The properties of the material can be adjusted depending on the fatty acid structure and the number of propylene glycol units inserted.

Esterified propoxylated glycerol (EPG) was patented by the Atlantic Richfield Company in 1986. The fatty acid components can be derived from naturally occurring or synthetic fatty acids or naturally occurring oils, including soybean oil, olive oil, cotton seed oil, corn oil, tallow and lard. Depending on the choice of fatty acid, non-caloric fat substitutes with physical properties ranging from liquid oils through to fats and greases are the result. It is claimed that EPGs are essentially resistant to intestinal absorption and do not hydrolyse significantly in the digestive tract, possibly because of the secondary ester linkage.

With the ability to tailor the melting point and other functional properties, depending on the choice of fatty acids, the potential applications for EPGs are as broad as those for Olestra. Again, the potential concerns from a regulatory standpoint of exposure to such quantities of a novel, poorly digested material will arise. The potential also for anal leakage and for the removal of fat-soluble vitamins must also exist with this material in a similar way to Olestra.

5.3.2.3 Polysiloxane. Polysiloxane is an organic derivative of silica with a linear polymeric structure (Frye, 1986). Polysiloxane can be an organic radical such as all methyl, or partly methyl and partially phenyl groups. These polymeric compounds are chemically inert, non-absorbable and claimed to be non-toxic. They are stable and maintain their viscosities over a wide range of temperatures, resistant to oxidation, hydrolysis and degradation, and are similar in their solubility characteristics to non-polar lipids. Phenyl methyl polysiloxane is an oil with properties close to that of soybean oil. It has a lipid-like character with respect to its behaviour in organic solvents and it is this material that has been studied as a potential fat substitute. A patent has been granted to Dow Corning Corporation.

Feeding trials in rats have demonstrated that polysiloxane has the potential to assist in weight reduction. Animals on a polysiloxane diet lost more weight than controls despite having similar food intakes. These results suggest absorption of caloric substances derived from partial digestion. No compensation for the caloric dilution with polysiloxane was observed. There appears to have been little work with the safety of these materials and the state of their development is probably not very advanced.

Applications for polysiloxanes have been claimed by Dow Corning to be peanut butter, mayonnaise, popcorn, salad dressings and baked products. This material is thus quite versatile in its potential applications, but it is another potential fat substitute which is unlikely to be developed to the point of commercialisation.

5.3.2.4 Glycerol dialkyl ethers. Glycerol dialkyl ethers have been patented by Swift and Company (Trost, 1981). Careful choice of alcohol allows the functonal characteristics of the fat substitute to be controlled. These materials are essentially non-absorbable and non-digestible. Again, and in a similar way to those other fat substitutes described earlier, these materials are claimed to be versatile in their potential applications. However, little additional information has appeared in the literature and so their state of development is probably not very advanced.

5.3.2.5 Polycarboxylic esters. A patent issued to CPC International describes a low-calorie fat substitute derived from stable polycarboxylic acids with two-four polycarboxylic acid groups containing straight or branched carbon chains of between 8 and 30 atoms. A patent along similar lines issued to Frito Lay Inc. describes fatty alcohol derivatives of malonic acid (Hamm, 1984).

Trialkoxytricarballyate (TATCA) is a clear, colourless oil prepared and evaluated as a potential fat substitute. Synthesis is effected under solvent-free conditions with an excellent yield. Interestingly, TATCA melts with polymorphic behaviour and in a manner similar to that of corn oil. It has greater viscosity than that of corn oil but is in the same range, and there is no notable difference in handling or pourability. It is claimed that TATCA is resistant to enzymic hydrolysis in the gut and hence little caloric value can be derived from this material. Apparently, there is low tolerence to the laxative effects that have been observed. Anal leakage occurs and the safety of TATCA is considered open to question.

Structurally TATCA resembles a triglyceride and so may be used in most vegetable oil applications including as a shortening, in butters, salad dressing and industrial frying oils. Although functionally it appears to be a versatile material, the safety problems that have been referred to are likely to preclude its development.

Trialkoxycitrate (TAC) can be synthesised from oleyl alcohol, although the yield is apparently low at only about 20%. Similarly to TATCA, TAC is a clear colourless oil and is composed mainly of fatty alcohol esters of citric acid. Thermal behaviour of TAC is similar to that of TATCA with polymorphism being exhibited. Viscosity, surface tension and sensitivity to enzymic hydrolysis are also similar to those of TATCA. Apparently, TAC does not have the thermal stability that TATCA exhibits and therefore cannot be used in frying-type applications, although it is claimed to be suitable for mayonnaise. Again, this material seems to no more than a curiosity and is unlikely to be developed on a commercial scale.

5.3.2.6 Other fat substitutes.   A number of other alternative fat-like products are under development or are in use. For instance, one under development by Dallas-based Frito-Lay is dialkyl dihexadecylmalonate (DDM), a non-caloric fatty alcohol ester of malonic and alkylmalonic acids.

5.3.2.7 Conclusions.   At first sight, fat substitutes, such as those discussed in the previous pages, might be expected to be extremely interesting to the food product developer. The ability to tailor functional properties to mimic those of specific fats and oils, through judicious selection of fatty acids, coupled with a clear, unequivocal calorie value of 'zero', suggests these ingredients would have significant potential. Unfortunately, the reality has not been so encouraging.

There seems little doubt that these ingredients really are able to deliver to foods the functional characteristics required of a fat substitute. Also, they are demonstrably non-caloric. However, even though they are, from a primary physiological standpoint, inert, their secondary physiological effects (anal leakage and the 'leaching' of fat-soluble vitamins) make their sanction by regulatory agencies difficult.

There have been a number of consequences of this unfulfilled promise. First, food manufacturers have ceased 'waiting' for these ingredients to appear on the statute books and have actively sought alternative routes to fat reduction in their products. Secondly, with a realisation that many of the approval problems of these fat substitutes stem directly from their 'zero-calorie' feature, other ingredients companies have sought to develop ingredients with similar functional characteristics, but which are partially metabolised. The advantage here has been to eliminate those problems which derive directly from the 'inertness' of fat substitutes. Finally, many ingredients have been developed and commercialised whose key functionality has been an ability to bind water. This characteristic is achieved in such a way that the ingredient plus water delivers some of the functional properties of the fat or oil being replaced, but at a much reduced energy contribution.

5.3.3 'Lower' calorie fat substitutes

5.3.3.1 Introduction. The concept of developing a metabolisable ingredient, capable of delivering fat/oil functionality, while also delivering a reduced energy value relative to the fat/oil being replaced, is new. The impetus for these developments came from the previously mentioned problems associated with fat substitutes, as well as the restricted versatility of fat replacers based on starches, proteins and hydrocolloids. Despite the relative 'newness' of this approach to fat replacement, some promising developments have been made. Some of the more interesting are now reviewed.

5.3.3.2 Carboxy/carboxylate esters. A patent was granted to Nabisco Brands Inc. in 1987 (Finley, 1987) describing the preparation and properties of low-calorie fat mimetics comprising carboxy/carboxylate esters (CCE).

This innovative development has been supported by a major research and development effort within Nabisco, at least judging by the number of patents which have issued. The key thrust of the development depends on the carboxy- and caboxylate residues attached to the carbon backbone offering differential reactivity with respect to cleavage by digestive enzymes. This results not only in the controlled and limited availability of energy, but also the selective conversion of the fat substitute to a product or intermediate with a less oil-like nature. The more readily digestible carboxylic acid residue can be a highly desirable essential fatty acid or a nutritionally advantageous carboxylic acid such as oleic, linolenic or eicosapentaenoic acid. Additionally, low molecular weight carboxylic acids, e.g. acetic, propionic, butyric, and so on may act as substituents, thus limiting caloric delivery and providing additional ability to control functionality.

The consequence of a product like this being 'controlled' in its degree of digestibility ensures that it is less likely to exist in the gastrointestinal tract as a persistent oil. This obviously will have benefits since there would be little tendency for anal leakage to occur. As has been noted, this is a potential problem with the consumption of Olestra and, in addition, there is probably less likelihood of fat-soluble vitamins being stripped out of the body.

The fatty acids and alcohols used to make these carboxy/carboxylate esters can be selected to achieve the desired texture and melt characteristics. The esters can be blended with each other or with triglyceride fats or even with sucrose polyester. The final product is partially, but not totally, broken down by the body. One of the consequences is that problems associated with non-metabolisable fat substitutes will be reduced and hence the safety prognosis should be substantially more straightforward.

The applications of these esters as disclosed in the Nabisco patent are extremely broad and cover all market sectors of the food industry where the products contain fats. This includes frozen desserts, puddings, pie fillings, margarine, flavoured spreads, mayonnaise, dressings, dairy products, dips, fats and oils, meat products, frostings, icings and confectionery.

Just as the potential applications of Olestra are equally broad, these products will also suffer from the potential regulatory problem which will result from the high levels of consumption that might occur. In a sense, the extreme versatility of these materials is in fact a drawback to their approvability.

5.3.3.3 Caprenin.

Procter and Gamble have also recently launched caprenin, developed in a joint venture with Grindsted Products. Caprenin is a reduced-calorie fat, with functional properties similar to cocoa butter.

It differs structurally from most fats in that two of its fatty acids are unsaturated medium chain acids, caprylic (C_8) and capric (C_{10}), and the third is behenic acid (C_{22}). Caprylic and capric acids are obtained from coconut and palm kernel oils, whereas behenic acid is found in peanuts, some marine oils and hydrogenated rapeseed oil. The combination of behenic acid, which is only partially absorbed by the body, and the medium chain acids, which are metabolised like carbohydrates, yields a fat with 5 kcal g^{-1}.

According to Procter and Gamble, caprenin is targeted at markets such as soft candies and confectionery coatings for fruits, nuts and cookies. These markets have been targeted because caprenin is claimed to provide the rich, creamy and chocolatey taste of cocoa butter. Early this year, Procter and Gamble began selling caprenin to M&M Mars for use in candy bars. In Spring 1992, M&M Mars launched a reduced-calorie bar product called Milky Way II. This product, in a test market in a small number of locations in the USA, contains 25% fewer calories than the standard Milky Way bar. Its market success is not yet assured, but it must be regarded as something of a technical triumph. Although caprenin is a key ingredient, the calorie claim also relies on incorporation of polydextrose, Pfizer's bulk sugar replacement ingredient. Caprenin was launched on the basis of an assumption of generally recognised as safe (GRAS) status, but Procter and Gamble have now filed a petition with FDA to affirm caprenin's status as GRAS.

One of the important features of this development is that it is, in basic concept, very similar to the carboxy/carboxylate esters development of Nabisco. The key difference appears to be that regulatory clearance of caprenin is unnecessary. Thus, it has to be possible that by the time Nabisco's development is on the statute books, caprenin (and other similar ingredients) will have a firm lock on this sector of the market.

5.3.3.4 Neobee M-5.   Another, similar product, under development by Stepan Corporation of Northfield, Illinois, is Neobee M-5, a medium chain triglyceride (MCT), containing fatty acids obtained from mixed triglycerides in coconut oil.

Although only about 1 kcal g^{-1} less than a typical fat, MCTs are metabolised more like carbohydrates, and are burned for energy rather than stored. A drawback of MCTs is that, when hydrolysed, the resulting free fatty acids have an 'off' flavour that is difficult to mask. At this point, it is also not known whether these, and other alternative fats, will be considered as fats and count as 'total' grams of fats and 'calories from fat' on food labels.

5.3.3.5 Conclusions.   Developments of this type are intellectually satisfying. They have been borne out of an understanding that the functional demands of fats/oils are such that only a versatile fat substitute can hope to find really broad application, coupled with an appreciation that approval of a zero-calorie fat substitute is unlikely. Providing this sort of ingredient can be made at costs which are acceptable within the normal framework of food product development, they must be anticipated to make significant contributions to the development of lower fat food products.

5.3.4 *Carbohydrates as fat replacers*

5.3.4.1 Introduction. Ingredients such as modified starches and gums, when combined at the optimum levels, can offer some reduction in fat content in foods due to their ability to bind water, provide texture and viscosity/consistency. Many starches and modified starches with similar functional characteristics, capable of replacing some fat/oil in selected products are now commercially available. Generally, these products are only suitable for use in foods which normally contain some water; they are not suitable for 'solid' foods such as biscuits or snacks.

Although it would be possible to provide a catalogue of these starches, because there are few if any technical differences between many of them, the discussion which follows will simply review the characteristics of selected ingredients which have received the most media attention and are quite well established in the market.

5.3.4.2 Paselli SA2. Paselli SA2 was developed and is marketed throughout the world by Avebe of Holland. It is a partially hydrolysed potato starch product with a dextrose equivalent (DE) of about five. It is produced by a gentle enzymic hydrolysis of the long chain amylose and amylopectin fractions.

At concentrations greater than 20% in aqueous systems, Paselli SA2 forms a thermoreversible gel. The texture of this gel is similar in many respects to that of fat or oil. Paselli SA2 can be dissolved in aqueous systems by homogenisation or by heating and stirring at between 50 and 100°C. In food processing, dry Paselli SA2 is preferably mixed with other dry ingredients to ensure a uniform mixture. The dry mixture is then added to the aqueous ingredients of the formulation. Within a short time, solutions containing more than 20% of Paselli SA2 begin to form white gels with fat-like textures. Although the ultimate strength of the gel will be reached after approximately 4 days in most applications, final gel setting effectively is realised within 24 hours. The strength of the gel will depend on the pH and temperature at which the starch is hydrated, but it is stable over a broad range of pH conditions. Maximum gel strength is obtained between pH 3.5 and 5.0. The thermoreversible nature means that the gel will melt on heating above about 50°C giving a low-viscosity solution, but this solution will form a gel again when it is cooled. The gel also forms a stable mixture with fat and oil products and is claimed to mix easily with other ingredients.

Being a starch-derived carbohydrate material, it will deliver a caloric value of 4 kcal g^{-1}, but in normal application it is typically used at around a 25% concentration, meaning that its effective caloric value is only 1 kcal g^{-1}. This compares with the 9 kcal g^{-1} of the fat or oil replaced.

Although Paselli SA2 is claimed to have broad versatility in food formulations, in reality its applications are largely restricted to those which contain relatively high concentrations of water. This is an inevitable consequence of the fact that its optimum functionality is found when it is used at a concentration in water of around 25%. Thus its applications are mainly restricted to what can be broadly termed as 'liquid emulsion' systems such as mayonnaise, salad dressings, spreads and desserts. For example, the manufacturers recommend that Paselli SA2 can be used in mayonnaise and dips, that it adds body and creaminess to soups and sauces and that it makes bakery fillings and creams thicker and smoother. It is also claimed to enhance the creaminess of dairy products such as desserts and toppings, as well as to find some applications in meat and sausage products.

5.3.4.3 N'Oil. N'Oil was developed and is marketed by the National Starch and Chemical Corporation of New Jersey, USA. It is a tapioca dextrin which is claimed to replace fat or oil partially or totally in selected food products. N'Oil is prepared by heating tapioca starch in the presence of hydrochloric acid. This treatment degrades the starch, reduces the viscosity of the cooked starch dispersion and leads to the formation of gels. Conversion to a DE of less than five is sufficient and National Starch suggest that the preferred product will have a DE of two or less.

N'Oil is available as a free flowing white to off-white powder and, like Paselli SA2, is able to form thermally reversible gels which are claimed to have fat-like organoleptic properties and will also form intimate mixtures with fats and oils in food systems. Gels are formed at concentrations in excess of 20% in water and they also melt at temperatures between 50 and 100°C.

National Starch has now developed a family of fat replacer ingredients, targeted primarily at different food applications.

5.3.4.4 C*Pur 01906 and C*Pur 01907. Cerestar have developed two low-DE potato maltodextrins which can achieve high-fat reductions. This is possible due to the ability of these maltodextrins also to form thermo-reversible fat like gels.

Both these maltodextrins are made by the enzymic conversion of potato starch. After spray drying, the conversion process results in free flowing white powders with a moisture content of less than five percent. These products differ in their degree of hydrolysis, expressed by a slightly higher DE value with C*Pur 01907 (3–5, compared with DE 2–5 for C*Pur 01906). While this difference provides products of similar carbohydrate composition, the gel strength in solution varies significantly. The difference in gel strength between the two maltodextrins is most clear at concentrations of 15 and 20%. At these concentrations, C*Pur 01907 yields a 'soft gel', whereas C*Pur 01906 gives 'hard gels'. The gel strengths of both products show no significant differences, indicating suitability in a diverse range of food systems ranging from acidic salad dressings to 'neutral' dairy and meat systems (Lawson, 1991).

5.3.4.5 Other starch-based fat replacer ingredients.   There are now many newly launched starch-based fat replacer ingredients on the market. For example, National Starch has now added four other replacer ingredients to their portfolio, each of which is targeted at a particular product sector of the food industry.

AE Staley brought out Stellar in 1992, which is somewhat different from the previously described starches in that it is a 'microcrystalline' starch (Anon, 1992). It forms a 25% solids cream when sheared with water and is also designed to replace fat or oil on a 1:1 basis. Thus, in application terms it is similar to the Paselli SA2 and N'Oil products. Interest from the food industry has, to date, been principally from within the meat products, dressings and frozen dessert sectors.

All of these fat replacers suffer from the limitation that they must be hydrated or 'functionalised' prior to incorporation into foods. Although food manufacturers are able to accommodate with relative ease the additional processing necessary, there has been some reluctance on the part of some manufacturers to introduce process changes.

5.3.4.6 Conclusions.   There are many starch-derived ingredients which are purported to replace the characteristics of the fat or oil being replaced. While there are food products amenable to this technology, the range is limited by the requirement that most suitable foods must contain water. Without that, the necessary functionality for the ingredient cannot develop. Thus, although these replacer ingredients have had quite an important impact on selected product sectors, their versatility is limited and this must be acknowledged.

5.3.5 Proteins as fat replacers

5.3.5.1 Introduction.   Protein-based fat replacer ingredients are, in function, similar to the modified starch ingredients already described. Their ability to bind water while delivering the texture and mouthfeel of fat or oil determines whether or not they will function satisfactorily.

5.3.5.2 Simplesse.   The protein-based fat replacer which has received the most publicity is without question 'Simplesse' from the NutraSweet Company. Simplesse was affirmed as GRAS by the US Food and Drug Administration early in 1990.

In concept, it is similar to the microcrystalline starch (Stellar) from AE

Staley. It too is 'microparticulated', though in contrast to Stellar, it is based on egg white and/or milk proteins. The protein is processed using heat and high shear, thus generating protein particles that are microscopic in size. These microparticles are roughly spheroidal. High shear heat processing is followed by a series of steps that may include ultrafiltration, dry blending of ingredients, hydration with water and pH adjustment with food grade acids, bases or both. Other steps may include deaeration and heat pasteurisation.

Initially, the approved use of Simplesse was as a thickener or texturiser for frozen dessert-type products. Early problems with frozen dessert product shrinkage have now been overcome. Subsequently, approved applications have been extended and Simplesse is in a variety of foods including low-fat cheeses, low-fat margarine spreads, and dairy desserts as well as low-fat frozen desserts (Singer *et al.*, 1991, 1992).

5.3.5.3 Lita. Other protein-based fat replacers are also in development. A zein-based product, called Lita, is under development by Enzytech Food Ingredients in the USA. When hydrated, Lita apparently simulates the sensory and physical characteristics of an oil-in-water emulsion. This is due to the Lita protein microspheres having approximately the same dimensions (0.3–3 microns) and spherical shape as the oil droplets found in dairy cream or other oil-in-water food emulsions.

A number of reasons for selecting zein as the protein base have been claimed:

1. Zein is naturally hydrophobic because of a high incidence of non-polar amino acids. As a result, zein does not need thermal denaturation to be capable of microparticulation.
2. Zein has ethanol/water solubility properties which mimic most fats and are unlike most proteins.
3. Zein is derived from (GRAS) corn gluten.
4. Zein is naturally present as spherical bodies *in situ*.
5. Raw material costs are low. Corn gluten is inexpensive (about $0.14/lb) and contains about 30–35% zein.

One drawback is that highly purified zein must be used since it has a tendency to associate with other compounds that are strongly flavoured. Enzytech claim to have developed a purification process which achieves an 'unprecedented' level of purity, and indicate market targets broadly in line with those for Simplesse and the starch-based fat replacers.

5.3.5.4 Conclusions. As noted earlier, these ingredients are functionally similar to the starch-derived equivalents. Thus, they confer similar benefits, as well as suffering from the same technical limitations. Nonetheless, they are 'label-friendly' ingredients, and so will find industry willing to use them, should their performance prove satisfactory.

5.3.6 Fat replacer formulations

5.3.6.1 Introduction.   There is now quite a range of formulated ingredients available which are targeted to replace fat and oil in selected products. In performance, they resemble the modified starches and proteins already described. They are usually composed of food materials already consumed as part of the food supply, and this familiarity to industry offers certain attractions. Generally, their ability to replace fats and oils mimics that of the modified starches and proteins. They, too, depend for their functionality on an ability to bind water, while delivering the appropriate sensory characteristics.

5.3.6.2 Microcrystalline cellulose.   Microcrystalline cellulose (MCC, cellulose gel) is a non-fibrous form of cellulose in which the plant cell walls have been broken into fragments ranging in size from 25 microns to less than 1 micron. Only the physical form of the cellulose raw materials is changed in the course of the manufacture of MCC; cellulose in fibre form is converted to cellulose in particle form. These crystalline cellulose particles are then combined with carboxymethyl cellulose to produce a colloidal cellulose gel, marketed by FMC Corporation. MCC serves as a protective colloid and allows aqueous dispersion of the cellulose microcrystals from a dry powder form.

The colloidal grades of MCC are highly functional food ingredients in aqueous systems. On proper dispersion, the cellulose crystalites set up a three-dimensional network with particles less than 0.2 microns. It is the formation of this insoluble network, held together by weak hydrogen bonds, that gives these colloidal materials their functional properties.

The colloidal dispersion is highly thixotropic, temperature stable, and adds body, while imparting a clean mouthfeel. The gels contribute no calories to foods in which they are incorporated. Applications include frozen desserts, salad dressings, whipped toppings and mayonnaises.

5.3.6.3 Slendid.   Slendid, from Hercules, is pectin whose gelling with calcium is induced under conditions of shear. The shearing 'shreds' the gel into small particles, which consist of more than 95% water, and have a fat-like appearance, texture and mouthfeel. It is claimed that Slendid is able to replace up to 100% of the emulsified fat in products.

5.3.6.4 Veri-Lo.   This year, Pfizer began marketing a fat extender called Veri-Lo. Using a proprietary emulsion system in water, the fat-containing product forms gel particles. The particles are about the size of typical fat globules and fat coated so that Veri-Lo is perceived to taste and behave like fat while offering significant calorie reductions. Veri-Lo is a GRAS product intended for low temperature applications such as mayonnaises, sauces, dressings and dairy foods. It is sold in two ready-to-use forms for replacing 67 to 75% of fat. Veri-Lo 100 contains 33% soybean oil with 3.1 cal g^{-1}. Veri-Lo 200 contains 25% milk fat and 2.3 cal g^{-1}. Pfizer's products are a compromise between the flavour that fat contributes and fat reduction. Others in the industry acknowledge that making products without fat is difficult and that many may have serious flavour defects. Some even suggest that small amounts of fat, qualifying for low-fat rather than fat-free standards, may creep back into foods to deliver better tasting products to somewhat disenchanted consumers.

5.3.6.5 Conclusions.   These formulations all depend, in part, on the use of 'structured water' to deliver the appropriate functionality. Thus, they too are identical in concept to the modified starches and proteins already described. They are frequently comprised of ingredients with which manufacturers and consumers are familiar, and this is marketed to advantage. One additional advantage of formulated products is that their properties are easier to tailor to specific food sectors; they offer more flexibility than is frequently the case with single component fat replacer ingredients.

5.3.7 Sensory implications of fat reduction

Changing the fat content of foods can have a profound impact on sensory characteristics. This has further implications on consumer preference and food choice.

Current research suggests that the role of fat in foods (in this context) is to 'round' the characteristic flavour notes. This is thought to be a consequence of one or more of the following mechanisms:

(i) the background flavour of the lipid components of the fat may have a modulating effect on the other flavours;
(ii) the mouthcoating effect of fats may have an effect on the availability of flavour components to the appropriate oronasal receptors;
(iii) the partitioning of flavour components between fat and oil phases in the food will modulate release of flavour components during the process of mastication.

These last two processes may be manifested in different temporal characteristics of flavour perception in the mouth. Consequently, the flavouring of reduced and no-fat foods is not a straightforward process. Many flavour companies have recognised this and are developing flavours specifically for these foods which aim to restore the sensory character of the full-fat equivalent.

5.4   Markets for fat-reduced foods and fat replacer ingredients

5.4.1   Introduction

Food manufacturers continue to be under pressure to satisfy consumer demands for reduced-fat foods. Consequently, food ingredient companies, responding to the apparent opportunity presented by these consumer demands, are striving to develop new ingredients which will effectively replace fat in foods. However, fat reduction is not a new objective, nor is it an objective littered with failure, for the food manufacturing industry has had a long record of success in satisfying consumer demands for fat-reduced foods in many significant market sectors.

Consequently, and in the light of these observations, it is sensible for food and ingredient manufacturers alike to look carefully at the current markets for fat-reduced foods and fat replacer ingredients. Careful analysis is needed to put some perspective on the real size of the opportunity for fat replacer ingredients by product sector and to avoid falling into the trap of believing there will necessarily be a substantial market for all ingredients delivering a fat-like functionality.

To illustrate the potential for ingredient manufacturers to be misled into believing there is huge potential for fat replacer ingredients, it is merely necessary to consider the success of fat-reduced dairy products, most of which has been achieved without recourse to using fat replacer ingredients. In the UK in 1990, lower fat milks had one third of the total milk market. All of this market was satisfied without using fat replacers, for simply by removing all or a portion of the fat from milk to give skimmed or semi-skimmed versions presents consumers with a satisfactory alternative. In this case, of course, there is no market for any of the many fat replacer ingredients available.

Other product sectors are similarly satisfied by use of simple and/or innovative technology. For example, emulsifiers and stabilisers have been developed specifically for low-fat spread products, none of which is described as 'fat replacer', even though their function is to maintain the integrity of lower fat versions. Many lower fat meat products have been made available which merely rely on the use of lean meat in place of fat. While it is true that this is an expensive route to meeting the product target, it has proved to be a relatively simple solution.

These examples should serve to illustrate the potential which undoubtedly exists for wild exaggeration of market estimates for fat replacer ingredients. The message here is undoubtedly that companies should avoid being seduced by the media hype, and focus on providing solutions to the key product issues of the day.

5.4.2 Markets for fat-reduced foods

Data on the markets for fat-reduced foods are principally available from the USA market. Although the extents of market shares achieved within particular food categories vary by country, the trends in the USA show an impressive uniformity of steady growth.

Data gathered by the A.D. Little Company for 1989 (Rudolph, 1991) illustrate clearly the market shares (%), market values ($) and growth trends, by product sector. These data are presented in Table 5.3. These data can be further summarised (Table 5.4) to illustrate both the current value of the reduced fat/calorie market, and also the scope that must exist for growth. Realisation of this growth will depend, of course, on the availability of ingredients capable of requiring few if any compromises by the consumer.

Clearly, with the reduced-fat/reduced-calorie sector merely accounting for less than 10% of the total market, there must be tremendous scope for market expansion in this area. This statement can be justified by considering the parallel example of low-calorie or diet beverages. In the carbonated sector, these now account for more than one third of the total carbonates market. The products deliver sensory experiences virtually indistinguishable from those delivered by the sugar sweetened standards, and so when it becomes possible, through ingredient developments, to offer the consumer similarly indistinguishable nutritionally modified versions, significant market growth must be anticipated.

Table 5.3 Market size for reduced-fat/low-calorie products in the USA in 1989

Food category	Market share (%)	Total value ($ million)	Growth trend (+/−; %)
Mayonnaise/ Spoonable dressings	23	1342	+13
Pourable dressings	27	933	+11–13
Margarines/spreads	33	2177	+22

Bakery
    Breads
    Sweet
	4.9
	2.0 }
		19 495	>15

Processed meats	<5	17 040	?
Icings/frostings	<5	192	?
Processed cheese	3	2317	+22
Frozen desserts	26	5698	+5–10
Cake mixes	<10	504	?
Snack foods	<5	9400	?

Table 5.4 Summary of USA market for reduced-fat/reduced-calorie foods in 1989

Food category	Market size ($ million)	Reduced-fat/reduced-calorie market
Mayonnaise/salad dressings	1324	309
Pourable salad dressings	933	250
Margarines and spreads	2177	720
Ice cream/frozen desserts	5698	1482
Processed cheese	2317	133
Processed meats	17 040	850
Bakery products	19 495	1600
Cake mixes	504	50
Icings and frostings	192	2
Snack foods	9400	470
Totals	59 098	5 866

5.4.3 Markets for fat replacer ingredients

Although the market value share for fat-reduced foods is just less than 10% of the total market value in the USA, the fat-reduced market is still significant in size and of really interesting potential for food ingredient manufacturers. However, as has already been mentioned, there are a variety of formulation and processing techniques available to manufacturers to reduce fat levels in many foods without resorting to the use of what are marketed as fat replacers. The consequences of this are clearly illustrated by data from Industrial Market Research International (Seisun, 1992) which show that the value of sales for fat replacer ingredients in 1991 was only around $60 million (Table 5.5).

5.5 Conclusions

It is clear that the food industry is working hard to meet consumer demands for fat-reduced foods, but that the current limitation on market growth is due to a shortage of suitable ingredients. Ingredient manufactur-

Table 5.5 Fat replacer market values

Fat replacer	Market value ($ million)	Share of total (%)
Hydrocolloids	52.5	87
Proteins	7.0	12
Other	1.0	1
Total	60.5	100

ing companies are trying to fill the gap, but some of the technical and regulatory issues they confront militate against rapid progress on either front. Therefore, there has been a tendency for food manufacturers to launch products which are unable to deliver sufficient quality to consumers, and so these products have failed. What industry should guard against now is the possibility that these failures to meet quality demands will simply turn consumers away from the concept of fat-reduced foods. To some extent, this scenario has already happened with 'added fibre' food products. Consumers proved willing to embrace this concept with real enthusiasm, but failure to deliver products of sufficient quality, virtually destroyed the market opportunity.

Providing industry is prepared only to launch foods which are of good quality, there is no reason why the markets for fat-reduced foods and the ingredients on which many products will depend should not develop rapidly. Published estimates suggest that the market for low-fat foods will grow to $10–15 billion by 1994, showing a growth rate of 10–15% each year over the next five years. If these estimates prove accurate, both food ingredient and food product manufacturers will reap significant rewards throughout the 1990s.

References

American Heart Association (1978) Diet and coronary heart disease. *Circulation*, **58**, 762A–765A.

Anon (1992) Shear simplicity reduces fat. *Prepared Foods*, June, 77.

Finley, J. (1987) Carboxy/carboxylate esters as fat replacer ingredients. *European Patent Application*, 303,523.

Frye, C.L. (1986) Fat and oil replacements as human food ingredients. *European Patent Application*, 205,273.

Hamm, D.J. (1984) Preparation and evaluation of trialkoxycarballylate, trialkoxycitrate, trialkoxyglycerylether, jojoba oil and sucrose polyester as low calorie replacements of edible fats and oils. *J. Food Sci.*, **49**, 419–428.

Haumann, B.F. (1986) Getting the fat out. *J. Am. Oil Chem. Soc.*, **63**, 278–288.

Lawson, P. (1991) Use of carbohydrates as fat replacers. *Food Ingredients Proc. Internat.*, January 17–21.

McCormack, C. (1991) American perceptions of low calorie products. In: *The Future for Low Calorie Sweeteners in the European Community and Eastern Europe*. Proceedings of the 1991 ISA Annual Conference. CPL Press, Newbury, UK, pp. 48–62.

Rudolph, M. (1991) Fat substitutes – A U.S. perspective. In: *Fat Substitutes*. Proceedings of a symposium held at the Leatherhead Food RA, England, November, 1990, pp. 22–51.

Seisun, D. (1992) Quantifying the current and potential market for fat reduction and low-fat foods. In: *Fat and Cholesterol Reduced Foods*. Proceedings of the third annual IBC Conference, New Orleans, U.S.A.

Senauer, B., Asp, E. and Kinsey, J. (1991). *Food Trends and the Changing Consumer*. Egan Press, St Paul, Minnesota, USA.

Singer, N., Latella, J. and Yamamato, K. (1991) Reduced fat yogurt. *US Patent*, 5,096,731.

Singer, N., Latella, J. and Yamamato, K. (1991) Reduced fat sour cream. *US Patent*, 5,986,730.

Trost, V.W. (1981) Low calorie fat substitutes. *Canadian Patent*, 1,106,681.

6 Fat and calorie-modified bakery products

R.L. BARNDT and R.N. ANTENUCCI

6.1 Introduction

Not long ago the terms 'low-fat', 'fat-free', 'cholesterol-free' or 'reduced-calorie' would not have applied to sweet bakery products. Today these products are becoming well known to the consumer as more and more baking establishments are offering 'healthier' alternatives. The present day consumer is struggling with the conflict between health and indulgence. This conflict is particularly strong in the baked goods segment since these products are typically made from whole milk, sugar, eggs and butter, major sources of fat, calories or cholesterol. How does the consumer cope with this conflict? Perhaps by becoming better informed about food choices and adopting a healthier diet and lifestyle. Today's consumer is changing consumption patterns which often means consuming sweet baked goods less often. And when baked goods are consumed, premium quality products are often selected to satisfy the craving for indulgence.

The baking industry has responded to changing consumption patterns with a wide variety of new product introductions designed to meet consumer demand for a healthier lifestyle. The range of healthier product choices includes modifications to fat, calories, cholesterol and sodium with most of the effort placed on fat and cholesterol elimination. Product modifications are achieved in part by new developments in ingredient technology. Resulting product quality has varied thus far. Improvements in overall quality will be dependent upon the skill and expertise of the master bakers and food scientists applying new ingredient technology to bakery products. The use of traditional ingredients such as whole milk, eggs and butter are being replaced by new variations of standard ingredients such as starches, fibers and gums. These ingredients are being used in a non-traditional fashion, as fat replacers or sparers. The role of sugar is being reduced through the use of low-calorie bulking agents such as polydextrose or fibres in combination with new heat stable, high-potency sweeteners like sucralose.

The fourth annual Prepared Foods research and development investment survey conducted in 1992 identified 'reduced-fat, reduced-calorie and diet foods' as the number one product development objective (Anon, 1992a). When industry segments were polled, 76% of the bakery, biscuit and cracker respondents indicated increased activity involving reduced-fat, reduced-calorie or diet food product development.

Consequently, this chapter will review recent developments regarding the formulation and marketing of fat and calorie-modified bakery products. The emphasis of this chapter will be on sweet baked goods rather than bread since the technology used in light bread manufacture is better documented than for sweet baked goods.

6.2 Marketing overview

6.2.1 Calorie Control Council United States consumer survey

The Calorie Control Council has conducted five surveys over the past 14 years designed to measure consumer attitudes and behavior in the United States. The most recent study was completed in January of 1991 and surveyed trends in dieting and the use of low-calorie, sugar-free and low-fat products. Earlier studies concentrated on sugar replacement since this has been the primary means of achieving low-calorie foods. However, with the emergence of low-fat products, this most recent study was the first to include information on low-fat products. Several of the survey findings are relevant to the baking industry and have bearing on the development of nutritionally modified bakery products. A summary of the key research findings was disclosed by Nabors (1992) and is discussed below.

First, approximately 141 000 000 Americans consume low- or reduced-calorie and/or fat products. Of this total, 124 000 000 Americans currently consume low- or reduced-fat foods and beverages. This includes 70 million women and 54 million men equivalent to 67% of the US adult population. From the magnitude of these numbers, it is obvious that consumers are taking measures to maintain their health, reduce fat and control caloric intake. An interesting fact is the usage of these low- and reduced-fat products by both female and male populations indicating broad-based consumer demand. This usage level has grown since earlier surveys.

It is not surprising that the most popular low-fat products were low-fat dairy products such as cheese, yogurt and sour cream (Table 6.1). However, 25% of adults and 37% of low-fat users consumed low-fat cakes, breads and other baked goods indicating strong consumer interest in this developing market segment.

The 1991 Calorie Control Council survey found that 101 million adult Americans consumed low-calorie, sugar-free foods and beverages. This represents an increase from 45% in 1986 to 54% of the 1991 US adult population and indicates a continuing strong consumer demand for low-calorie and sugar-free products. In recent years strong growth has occurred among men with the most dramatic increase among respondents age 60 and over. Given the demographics of the US population, the population

Table 6.1 Most popular reduced-fat products in the USA

Product	% Total population	% Low-fat consumers
Cheese/dairy products	49	74
Beverages	43	64
Ice cream/frozen desserts	34	51
Chips/snack foods	31	46
Cakes/baked goods	25	37
Dinner entrées	23	34

Source: Calorie Control Council 1991 National Survey

segment over 60 represents a significant market opportunity for low-fat and low-calorie products.

The most popular low-calorie products remain sugar-free carbonated soft drinks, consumed by 78% of low-calorie consumers and 42% of the total population (Table 6.2). Sugar-free cakes and cookies are consumed by 17% of low-calorie consumers and 9% of the total population. These survey figures indicate interest on the part of the consumer in reduced-fat and low-calorie baked goods and represent an opportunity for the baking industry to develop this market segment.

The Calorie Control Council survey investigated how and why people are using low-calorie products. When the respondents were asked 'how' they dieted, 95% said they cut down on high-calorie, high-fat foods such as dessert items. Use of low-fat foods and beverages was mentioned by 89%, exercise by 85%, and use of low-calorie foods and beverages by 82% of the people questioned. Clearly these responses suggest an avoidance of indulgent foods like sweet baked goods which are high in calories, fat and cholesterol. This trend would suggest an opportunity for the baked goods

Table 6.2 Most popular low-calorie products in the USA

Product	% Total population	% Low-calorie consumers
Sugar-free carbonated soft drinks	42	78
Sugar substitutes	31	57
Sugar-free gum, candy	28	51
Sugar-free pudding, gelatin	18	34
Sugar-free frozen desserts	15	27
Sugar-free yogurt	12	22
Sugar-free powdered drink mixes	12	21
Sugar-free cakes, cookies	9	17
Other low-calorie or 'light' Foods/beverages	24	45

Source: Calorie Control Council 1991 National Survey

industry to respond with low-fat and low-calorie versions of full-calorie favorites to support the consumer demand for light foods.

When asked 'why' they used low-calorie or light foods, the most frequent reason was to stay in overall better health followed by maintaining current weight. Maintaining an attractive physical appearance, weight reduction and refreshment or taste were the next most frequently cited reasons for using low-calorie products. These responses suggest that many people who are non-dieters are including low-calorie and low-fat products as mainstream product additions to their diet. However, only 43% of the respondents indicated taste as the reason for using light foods and beverages. Satisfying taste is always a key attribute for overall product acceptance and repurchase. Therefore, improving the taste of nutritionally modified foods and beverages remains a critical factor for success by the food industry, and particularly the baking community.

The Calorie Control Council survey demonstrates broad-based interest in low-calorie and low-fat food and beverage products by both dieters and non-dieters. A significant portion of the US population is already consuming low-fat baked goods in support of their light eating style. A significant growth opportunity exists for the baking industry provided good tasting, low-fat and low-calorie baked goods can be developed which satisfy consumer demands for 'healthier indulgent' foods.

6.2.2 Baked goods concept research

The Calorie Control Council survey was useful in identifying general trends in consumer demand for low-fat and low-calorie food and beverage products. However, this research did not focus specifically on baked products. To answer the question whether consumers are interested in the concept of reduced-calorie bakery products containing low-calorie sweeteners, McNeil Specialty Products Company conducted a baked goods concept test.

The test was conducted for McNeil in 1987 by Burke Marketing Research, a nationally known independent market research company. Three forms of bakery products were evaluated, pies and cookies by concept only, and cakes by concept and product evaluation. Concepts were prepared for each baked product positioning the product as having one third less calories than a full-calorie version with the same taste. The cake cell had 600 participants, the pie cell 175 participants, and the cookie cell 251 participants. Based on concept alone, the consumers exhibited a strong interest in all three reduced-calorie baked products (Table 6.3). The top two box scores, defined as 'definitely buy' and 'probably buy', were 55% for cakes, 62% for pies and 60% for cookies. When the brand name of a leading baked goods company was added into the cake concept, purchase intent was even higher. The top box score for 'definitely will buy' increased from 12% to 26% and the 'probably will buy' score remained steady at 42%. This significantly increased the top two box score purchase intent from 55% for unbranded cake to 68% for a branded cake indicating the value of brand equity.

The research explored the reasons why respondents liked the concepts. 'Low in calories' and 'good taste' were the key concept likes for the cake (Table 6.4). 'Texture', 'variety of flavors' and 'natural/not artificial' were frequently mentioned for all three concepts. This suggests that many consumers do not want caloric savings at the expense of good taste, texture and variety.

The next area explored was the interest in product replacement versus purchase in addition to the brand normally consumed. As seen in Table 6.5, there is strong consumer interest in replacing their current brand of baked products with products represented by the new concepts.

The success of this proposition depends greatly on how well the concept satisfies consumer expectations for caloric reduction, taste and texture. This was tested in the cake cell by allowing positive purchase intent participants to taste a sucralose sweetened reduced-calorie cake. The reaction to the cake after trial was outstanding (Table 6.6). Ninety percent of the participants remained positively committed to purchase after tasting the reduced-calorie cake (i.e. top two box). Even among consumers with a neutral or negative purchase intent towards the concept, most expressed positive purchase intent (54% top two box) after trial.

Both positive and neutral/negative concept panelists indicated that the cake outperformed expectations created by the concept. Of the original positive and neutral/negative purchase intent participants, 91% and 85%, respectively responded that the cake was better or about the same as expected. This finding suggests that the consumer may have preconceived negative ideas about the taste and textural quality of nutritionally modified bakery products.

Table 6.3 Baked goods concept research: concept purchase intent (%)

	Cake	Pie	Cookie
(Base: consumed in past 90 days)	(600)	(175)	(251)
Definitely buy	12 ⎱ 55	20 ⎱ 62	17 ⎱ 60
Probably buy	43 ⎰	42 ⎰	43 ⎰
Might/might not	33	31	28
Probably not	9	7	8
Definitely not	3	0	5

Important learning: consumers exhibited a strong interest in reduced-calorie baked products

Source: McNeil Specialty Products Company, 1987

Table 6.4 Baked goods concept research: concept product likes (%)

	Cake	Pie	Cookie
(Base: total per group)	(600)	(175)	(251)
Low in calories	73	69	66
Taste/flavor	40	19	18
Texture	23	27	27
Variety of flavors	18	34	26
Natural/not artificial	8	9	4

Important learning: low in calories and good taste were the key concept likes

Source: McNeil Specialty Products Company, 1987

Table 6.5 Baked goods concept research: product replacement or addition (%)

	Cake	Pie	Cookie
(Base: Definitely/probably buy)	(332)	(108)	(152)
Buy instead of another brand that normally eat	69	75	70
Buy in addition to another brand that normally eat	31	24	28
Don't know	1	1	2

Important learning: most users would replace their current brand

Source: McNeil Specialty Products Company, 1987

Table 6.6 Baked goods concept research: purchase intent after trial (%)

	Cake cell
(Base: positive to concept)	(97)
Definitely buy	52 ⎫
Probably buy	38 ⎬ 90
Might/might not	6 ⎭
Probably not	3
Definitely not	1

Important learning: reaction to the cake after trial was outstanding

Source: McNeil Specialty Products Company, 1987

In an attitude and usage study conducted in August of 1989 by McNeil Specialty Products Company, the importance of taste in reduced-calorie baked goods was examined. A base of 271 people who had eaten or purchased baked goods in the past 30 days were asked if they would be willing to sacrifice taste for caloric reduction.

Nearly a half (49%) would be 'willing to sacrifice some taste' while 51% would 'not be willing to sacrifice some taste'. These results suggest that taste will be a compelling motivational factor in driving consumer purchase intent.

In summary, this research demonstrates a strong US consumer interest in good tasting, nutritionally modified bakery products. However, caloric or fat reduction alone may not be sufficient to expand this category as consumers seem unwilling completely to compromise on taste.

6.2.3   Cake mix concept research

The emphasis on development of low-fat bakery products is an indication that the baking industry feels fat reduction is more important to consumers than sugar reduction. This is evidenced by the fact that all three major US cake mix brands, Betty Crocker®, Duncan Hines® and Pillsbury®, have introduced reduced-fat cake mixes. In these examples, the majority of fat is removed from the cake mix and the bulk often replaced with carbohydrate fillers. Pillsbury also cites a 33–40% calorie reduction on their reduced-fat cake mix packages. Therefore, McNeil Specialty Products Company commissioned Burke Market Research in 1991 to conduct concept research to test the impact of caloric reduction when added to reduced-fat light cake mix product concepts.

The study design contained monadic and direct preference concept cells which evaluated the concepts of a 94% fat-free box cake mix against a product 94% fat-free plus 33% fewer calories. The 94% fat-free cake mix concept represents commercial light cake mixes introduced in the US marketplace at the time of the concept research. Central location screenings were undertaken in eight geographically dispersed markets. Each test cell had 200 respondents who were female heads of household 18–65 years of age. Each respondent had purchased a cake mix product in the previous three months.

Monadically, the 94% fat-free and 94% fat-free plus 33% fewer calories concepts generated comparable top two box purchase intent scores. The 94% fat-free concept scored 23% for 'definitely will buy' and 47% for 'probably will buy'. The 94% fat-free plus 33% fewer calories concept generated a slightly higher top box score of 29% and a 'probably will buy' score of 41%. Therefore, on a monadic basis, both concepts were judged to be highly motivating ideas.

Direct preference measures indicated a strong overall (79%/13%) preference for concepts mentioning calorie reduction *and* fat reduction (94% fat-free plus 33% fewer calories) versus fat reduction alone (94% fat-free). The reasons given by the respondents for positive purchase intent were fat-free, taste/flavor and fewer calories.

This concept research suggests that there is US consumer demand for cake mixes with low-fat *and* fewer calories. Furthermore, consumers are motivated by significant fat and caloric reductions when reassured of good taste.

6.2.4 Market trends in the United States

A marketing intelligence report published in January 1992 (FIND/SVP, 1992) provides an excellent overview of the sweet baked goods marketplace. The report estimates that US retail sales of sweet baked goods totaled $11.9 billion in 1991. Wholesale bakers accounted for $7.1 billion in sales while the value of goods produced at the retail level totaled about $4.9 billion. The total sales of retail baked goods grew substantially from $8.6 billion in 1987 to $11.9 billion in 1991. This equates with a compound annual growth rate of 8.7%.

The FIND/SVP report discusses an ongoing market shift involving the loss of market share by wholesale bakers, including all of the leading brands, to sweet goods produced by retail bakers, especially supermarket in-store bakeries. The segment of retail baked sweet goods is the fastest growing among all product types. For example, comparing retail baked versus plant baked, dessert cakes grew at a compound annual growth rate of 15.9 and 12.1%, respectively, breakfast cakes and sweet rolls at 16.0 and 4.7%, respectively, dessert pies at 15.5 and 6.3%, respectively, and cookies at 12.6 and 4.3%, respectively. In this case, 'retail baked' refers to retail sale of goods baked at retail bakeries including in-store or freestanding, while 'plant baked' refers to retail sales of goods baked in wholesale bakeries.

The total US retail sales of 'premium sweet baked goods' has grown from $3.1 billion in 1987 to $4.4 billion in 1991 accounting for 37% of total retail sales. The premium segment is dominated by five major national bakers who have a 55% sales share of the market. A 28% market share is held by the Entenmann's® and Freihofer® brands belonging to Philip Morris's Kraft General Foods Corporation. Sara Lee®, Campbell Soup's Pepperidge Farm® and Kellogg's Mrs. Smith's® each have between 5 and 10% of the market. Another retailer worthy of mention is Heinz' Weight Watchers® with a 2% market share. The Weight Watchers brand is significant in the context of this chapter due to their historical development and marketing of sweet baked desserts targeted for health management. Entenmann's dominates the market for freshly baked cakes, coffee cake and sweet rolls. Pepperidge Farm dominates the market for premium cookies but Nabisco has made a move to capture some of the premium cookie business. Mrs. Smith's dominates the market for frozen pies. Sara Lee, Pepperidge Farm and Weight Watchers all compete to some extent in the frozen cake segment.

The FIND/SVP (1992) report noted that

the tactic of using real butter and whole eggs to establish a product as a premium product is becoming counterproductive. Butter and eggs are major sources of fat and cholesterol, and increasing numbers of consumers are trying to limit their fat and cholesterol intake. Although this trend is apparent in all socioeconomic strata, it is somewhat stronger among more affluent consumers, who are those most likely to purchase premium foods.

Thus the baking industry is faced with the problem of how to market traditionally indulgent foods to a marketplace concerned about intake of fats, sugar and cholesterol.

6.2.5 Projects lightning and thunder

How has the baking industry responded to consumer interest in nutritionally modified baked goods? They responded with a variety of new product introductions promoted as healthier versions of full-calorie baked goods. The predominate marketing theme has combined lower-fat or fat-free with cholesterol-free products. A review of one major baking company's contribution, the Entenmann's division of General Foods Bakery Companies, is warranted due to its role as a leader in fat-free baking technology.

The Entenmann's interest in fat-free bakery products took root in the autumn of 1987 (Malovany and Pacyniak, 1991). Gregory Murphy, a newly appointed president and chief executive officer of Entenmann's, suggested that they must be the first company to develop a fat-free, cholesterol-free product line with under 100 calories per serving. If this task were not difficult enough, an added requirement was that no product would be launched unless it matched Entenmann's historically high standards of quality at a reasonable cost. At that time, a fat-free product was considered revolutionary since the technology did not clearly exist to execute the concept. Therefore Entenmann's began a top secret program code named 'Project Lightning' to create a revolutionary and versatile technology that would replace fat in its entire bakery line.

Project Lightning combined the talents of master bakers who provided perspective on the art of baking with food scientists who contributed the ingredient technology. Together they attacked the problem of fat replacement by combining approaches from both a bakery ingredient and equipment perspective. It took roughly one and a half years of testing until the breakthrough technology was achieved. The technology involves the use of emulsifiers and hydrocolloids to replace the properties of fat in sweet bakery products. Entenmann's immediately began 'Project Thunder', the code name for the development of fat-free bakery formulas from the Project Lightning technology. The Project Lightning technology and Thunder formulas have been closely guarded by Entenmann's and are patent-pending.

By late 1989, Entenmann's had launched a line of fat- and cholesterol-free sweet baked goods. The initial line introductions included twelve varieties of loaf cakes, crunch cakes, cookies, coffee cakes and cheese pastries. The most difficult products to develop were cookies, due to the combination of high fat and low moisture. Sales for the fat-free line in the first full year were estimated at $200 million. For their efforts in developing and introducing the fat-free baking technology, Entenmann's received the 1990 Edison award for New Product Marketer of the Year from the American Marketing Association. Entenmann's was also awarded the grand prize for best retail product of the year at Gorman's New Product Contest.

6.2.6 How did the baking industry respond?

The introduction of the Entenmann's fat-free line was the impetus for other bakery companies to enter the US marketplace with fat-free and cholesterol-free products of their own. The following is an overview of how several major baking companies responded with product introductions into the US premium sweet baked goods marketplace.

At about the same time that Entenmann's launched their fat-free line, Charles Freihofer Baking Company launched a cholesterol-free line of cakes (FIND/SVP, 1992). Freihofer Baking is also a member of the General Foods Baking Companies and is a leading brand in the north eastern section of the United States.

Pepperidge Farm Division of Campbell Soup Company introduced the *Pepperidge Farm Dessert Light*® line in late 1989. The introductory line consisted of seven varieties of frozen cakes and desserts including single-serve items. The products have fewer calories (190 calories or less) and less sodium than full-calorie versions in their *American Collection*®. Some of the new varieties are lower in fat. In July 1991 they introduced a line of cookies low in total fat (17–28% fat range) and saturated fat, containing no cholesterol or tropical oils (Anon, 1991). The new brand is called *Wholesome Choice*® and complies with or exceeds the National Heart, Lung and Blood Institute's recommendation of a daily intake of 30% or less of calories from total fat. In mid-1992, the *Wholesome Choice* line represented 8–9% of the total Pepperidge Farm business (A.C. Nielsen Scantrack data, 1992).

In early 1990 Sara Lee introduced a new line of six single-serve frozen desserts, each with less than 200 calories (Liesse and Dagnoli, 1990). These products were launched nationwide under the *Sara Lee Lights*® brand name and contain about 33% fewer calories and are lower in cholesterol and sodium than a single serving of regular Sara Lee desserts. Nielsen Scantrack data for 1991 indicates that the *Lights* brand has captured a 5.6% unit share and 8.1% dollar share of the frozen dessert cake market.

Sara Lee followed the introduction of the *Lights* line with a *Free and Light*® single-serve line of 'healthy' frozen baked goods. This product line included pies, muffins, cakes, Danish and yogurt dessert items. The *Free & Light* line contains reduced-calorie products in the 70 to 170 calories per serving range which are also at least 98% fat-free, cholesterol-free and low in sodium. The introduction of the *Lights* and *Free & Light* product lines represented a departure from traditional indulgent desserts for which Sara Lee is well known. Throughout 1991, the *Free & Lights* product line held a 2.1% unit share and 2.4% dollar share of the total frozen coffee cake/sweet roll market (A.C. Nielsen Scantrack data, 1992).

Another major brand in the frozen bakery products category is *Weight Watchers International* by Heinz. The *Weight Watchers* brand responded to the market challenge by other major baking concerns by repositioning many of its products as 'healthy' rather than 'diet' foods (FIND/SVP, 1992). Many of their products were reformulated to reduce the level of fat, sodium and cholesterol. A review of Nielsen Scantrack data shows *Weight Watchers* to have a 10% unit share of the frozen cheesecake/dessert cake market, down from 13.2% in 1990. Their unit share in frozen coffee cakes/sweet rolls has grown from 3.8% in 1990 to 5.8% in 1991.

The Continental Baking Company, a subsidiary of Ralston Purina Company, introduced the *Hostess Lights*® line in 1990. The product line includes twelve muffin and coffee cake products as well as a light version of the famous Hostess Twinkie. The slimmed down version of the Twinkie has 110 calories per serving, is 94% fat-free and contains no cholesterol. The *Hostess Lights* line has experienced a slight increase in both fresh cake unit (3.4% vs. 3.2%) and dollar (5.9% vs. 5.7%) share in 1991 versus 1990 (A.C. Nielsen Scantrack data, 1992).

Nabisco is by far the US market leader in cookies and crackers. They have responded to consumer interest in healthier products with an increased effort to reduce fat and cholesterol in their cookie and cracker lines. Nabisco introduced a *Fat-Free Premium Cracker*® dropping the reference to saltine (Hess, 1990). The new cracker product has eliminated fat without the use of a fat substitute. In 1991, Nabisco introduced into the test market the *My Goodness*® line of healthy cookies (Dagnoli, 1991). The cookies obtain 30% of their calories from fat and are cholesterol-free. More recently, *Fat-Free Fig Newtons*® and *Fat-Free Apple Newtons*® were distributed nationally in early 1992 (Anon, 1992b). The fat-free Newtons are the first major cookie brand to be totally devoid of fat. The product utilizes egg whites as a substitute for shortening in the outer layer of the cookie. Thus far the fat-free varieties have been a big success. After only 22 weeks on the market, the new fig and apple varieties have already captured a 1.5% product share of the entire cookie category (A.C. Nielsen Scantrack data, 1992). The fat-free varieties have also provided incremental growth, in terms of product and dollar volume and share, to the entire Nabisco Newton line. Nabisco has also introduced the *SnackWell's*® line of low-fat and non-fat cookies and crackers.

Eli's, well known in the US for their cheesecake products, introduced a new light cheesecake under the *E'lites*® brand name. The product is 50% reduced in fat and 33% reduced in calories compared to their original cheesecake. *E'lites*® is the first baked good to use Simplesse, an all natural fat substitute, to enhance the creaminess of the product. In the US, three major brands dominate the cake mix category with over 90% unit share, *Betty Crocker* (General Mills), *Duncan Hines* (Procter and Gamble), and *Pillsbury* (Grand Metropolitan). Each has launched a light cake mix product in the 1990–1991 period. The light products have approximately an 8% unit and dollar share of the entire 1991–1992 cake mix category. This represents stronger growth than the full-calorie segment of the category, however, it is difficult to predict the success of these products at this early stage. The similarity in percent unit and dollar share suggests that these products are not premium priced versus full-calorie products. Historically, cake mixes have been a cost competitive category. This legacy makes it extremely difficult to introduce technologically advanced products (reduced-fat or reduced-calorie) with an inherently higher cost structure.

6.2.7 Calorie Control Council European consumer survey

The Calorie Control Council and Pfizer Specialty Chemicals Group collaborated on independent consumer research designed to determine current usage and attitudes towards low-calorie and reduced-fat products in Europe (Lemieux, 1992). Pfizer Specialty Chemicals Group initiated and funded the surveys. Booth Research Services was commissioned to conduct research in the United Kingdom, France and Germany. The survey interviewed a total of 1000 respondents in each country consisting of males and females of 18 years of age or older. The interviews took place in late 1991.

The results revealed that 64% of adults of age 18 or older in the three countries surveyed are consumers of low-calorie or reduced-fat products. This represents a total of approximately 81 million consumers purchasing light or healthier products. Of the 81 million, 30.5 million light consumers are in the United Kingdom, 31.5 million are in Germany, and 19 million consume light products in France. These segments represent significant portions of the total adult population in each country, 74% in the United Kingdom, 69% in Germany, and 48% in France. Thus a significant marketing opportunity exists for low-calorie products in Europe.

The survey identified the most popular low-calorie products. Sugar-free cakes and cookies were consumed by 5.3, 3.5 and 9.0% of the total population in the United Kingdom, France and Germany, respectively. This corresponds to 15, 13, and 19% of the low-calorie users in the United Kingdom, France and Germany, respectively. The European consumption figures compare favorably with consumption by low-calorie users (16.5%) and the total population (8.9%) in the United States.

When current low-calorie product users were asked if they had an interest in additional low-calorie products, nearly 60% responded favorably. Products which were mentioned most often included cookies, cakes and pies, indicating a strong consumer desire for a greater variety of low-calorie sweet baked goods.

The reasons Europeans use low-calorie products are similar to the reasons given by Americans: to 'stay in better overall health', to 'reduce sugar intake' and to 'maintain current weight'. Thus the theme of health management is a global trend. Furthermore, roughly 50% of the curent users of low-calorie products consume them on a daily basis. In France and Germany these products are consumed most frequently at breakfast while in the United Kingdom usage is most frequent at lunch and dinner. These trends contribute to a high frequency of purchase and help to identify the type of sweet baked goods which would be most successful in these countries.

The survey found that low-fat products are gaining popularity in each country. In the United Kingdom, 67% of adults consume low-fat products. In Germany, 53% consume low-fat products while France had the lowest consumption at 39% of adults. Table 6.7 compares the most popular reduced-fat products consumed in the United Kingdom, France and Germany against the products consumed in the United States. Dairy products and beverages head the list. Reduced-fat baked goods are consumed by 12% of the total population in the United Kingdom, 6% of the total population in France, and 19% of the total population in Germany. When these figures are converted to a low-fat user basis, 18% in the United Kingdom, 14.6% in France and 35% in Germany consume reduced-fat baked goods. These consumption estimates are lower than in the United States where approximately 25% of the total population and 37.4% of the low-fat users consume reduced-fat baked goods.

Table 6.7 Most popular reduced-fat products worldwide

	% Total population			
	UK	France	Germany	US
Margarine	54	22	40	N/A
Cheese/dairy	53	33	47	49
Beverages	35	11	33	43
Ice cream/frozen desserts	18	7	9	34
Crisps/snack foods	28	8	8	31
Dressings/sauces/mayonnaise	34	15	25	N/A
Baked goods	12	6	19	25
Dinners	14	13	13	23

Source: Calorie Control Council, 1991 European Survey
N/A = not available

The reasons cited for consuming low-fat products are similar to the reasons given for consuming low-calorie products, to 'stay in better overall health' and to 'reduce fat'. A significant percentage of the users expressed a desire for additional reduced-fat products with interest being highest in the United Kingdom and France. These consumer interests afford the baking industry an opportunity to grow this market segment through the introduction of high-quality, reduced-fat baked goods which satisfy European consumer demands.

6.2.8 International market trends

If the fat- and calorie-modified bakery product segment is in its early childhood in the United States, then this segment is in its infancy in the remainder of the world. The joint Calorie Control Council and Pfizer European survey identified tremendous interest in reduced-fat and low-calorie bakery products. However the consumption of these products in Europe is low compared to the United States. Presumably this is due to fewer nutritionally modified product options available to the European consumer compared to the American marketplace. Thus far, no major European baking company has taken the lead in producing nutritionally modified bakery products the way Entenmann's has in the United States.

In Canada a few bakery companies have ventured into the low-fat segment. A line of low-fat muffin mixes was introduced from Multifoods®, Loblaws® introduced a low-fat muesli muffin and Westons® introduced a line of low-fat coffee cakes. The Canadian approval of sucralose, a heat stable, high-potency sweetener, may stimulate the production of good tasting, low-calorie bakery products.

In Australia, a few well known names have entered the low-fat marketplace. White Wings®, a division of Goodman Fielder Wattie, has introduced a line of low-fat cake mixes and Sara Lee introduced a low-fat frozen cake line.

6.2.9 Cooking and baking in the home

Thus far the emphasis on healthier bakery products has been on retail product introductions by the baking industry. Attention now turns to how consumers can prepare healthier foods in their home, especially sweet baked goods which are lower in calories.

A significant opportunity exists for a good tasting, low-calorie sweetener that can be used in home cooking and baking applications to replace sugar. This is just one of the important findings from a table top sweetener attitude and usage study conducted for McNeil Specialty Products Company in 1991. Table 6.8 illustrates the ways in which sugar and low-calorie table top sweeteners are used most often. Addition to beverages is the most popular use for both sugar and low-calorie sweeteners. Cooking and baking is the second most popular use for sugar while low-calorie products are hardly used in this application. On a tonnage basis, 57% of the sugar volume used in the home goes into cooking and baking applications in contrast to only 1% of the low-calorie sweetener volume. This usage trend is supported by the survey finding that a significant number of low-calorie sweetener users are likely to use sugar in their cooking and baking applications. This finding is due in part to the lack of a good tasting, heat stable, low-calorie sweetener available in a form suitable for cooking and baking in the home. The table top sweetener market is dominated by only a few popular brands. These brands are marketed in several forms. The packet form is the most popular in the US and Canada while tablets are widely used in Europe and Australia. To a lesser extent, bulk forms are available which are better suited to home cooking and baking applications than packets or tablets.

Popular saccharin-based products include the Sweet'N Low® and Sugar Twin® brands in the United States. Sweetex with Natriblend (a saccharin–aspartame blend) and Hermesetas Sprinkle Sweet® are product examples found in Europe. These brands are available in bulk forms suitable for use in home cooking and baking applications. Sweet'N Low has a bulk concentrate form which requires a special measuring spoon to equate sweetness to a sugar equivalency. Sugar Twin, Sweetex and Hermesetas have a bulk spoon-for-spoon form designed to measure and pour like sugar. The spoon-for-spoon concept permits easy replacement of sugar with an equal volume of the sugar substitute resulting in identical sweetness intensity. However, a problem which all saccharin-based sweeteners suffer from is the unpleasant aftertaste inherent in the sweetener. This results in poor overall sweetness quality in end use applications.

Aspartame-based products are represented around the world primarily by the NutraSweet Spoonful™, Equal or Egal Spoonful®, or Canderel Spoonful™ brand names. These products are available in bulk spoon-for-spoon form but are used predominately for beverage or sprinkle-on applications. The product label notes that 'a loss of sweetness will occur if used in prolonged cooking or baking'. The manufacturer suggests addition after the cooking process.

Table 6.8 Table top sweeteners: ways used most often (%)

	Sugar users	Low-calorie users
(Base: total sample)	(385)	(72)
Beverages	47	79
Cooking/baking	31	3
Spinkle-on	19	12

Source: McNeil Specialty Products Company, 1991 Tabletop A&U

Sucralose received its first regulatory approval in September 1991 in Canada. The sweetener is marketed under the Splenda® brand name and is available to the consumer in both packet and granular spoon-for-spoon table top forms. The latter table top product measures and sweetens spoon-for-spoon and cup-for-cup like sugar. The heat stable sweetener is suitable for replacing sugar in a wide variety of home cooking and baking applications. Low-sugar and sugar-free recipes using sucralose are available from the distributor.

Thus sugar substitutes offer the consumer a low-calorie alternative to ordinary table sugar. In 1991, all low-calorie sweeteners commanded only a 5% share and bulk spoon-for-spoon products less than a 1% share of the total table top sweetener unit volume. Clearly these spoon-for-spoon products are underdeveloped relative to sugar usage for home cooking and baking applications. Low-calorie table top sweeteners which combine product performance with good taste would seem to be a powerful motivator to consumers interested in good health and superior taste in the baked goods they prepare at home.

6.3   Technical overview

6.3.1   Reduced-calorie baked goods

Formulation and production of low-calorie baked goods require creative use of non-standard food ingredients that are not typically found in traditional bakery products. These ingredient replacements can effect the multiple ingredient interactions in baked goods which influence texture, stability, flavor and sweetness. The use of these reduced-calorie non-standard food ingredients greatly effects the chemical and physical characteristics of baked goods including flavor, grain and texture, richness, aeration, tenderness and stability. Caloric reduction in baked goods often requires a reformulation using various reduced-calorie ingredients to build in the desired properties of the finished baked goods. In addition, ingredient trials and experimental duplication are often required to understand these complex ingredient interactions.

6.3.2   Fat replacement in baked goods

Fat is normally the first target for caloric reduction because it contributes more than twice the calories of either protein or digestible carbohydrate. Fat levels can be effectively reduced in baked goods by using ingredients which either simulate the functionalities of fat and/or enhance these properties.

Fats and oils greatly effect the physical properties of baked goods, particularly in product preparation. Fat dispersion in bakery mixes tends to disrupt the continuity of the gluten chains that form when flour proteins become hydrated. This creates areas of weakness in the structure, resulting in a shorter textured baked goods (Cauvain, 1987). Fat also provides aeration during the mixing stage which is the basis of cake structure. In cookies, fats, shortening and emulsifiers provide tenderization, lubrication, shelf life preservation, aeration, control of fat crystal growth and reaction with wheat proteins to modify dough consistency. The partial replacement of these functionally active baking ingredients with poly-dextroses, fibers and emulsifiers can produce acceptable cookies with the desired calorie reduction.

Fat functionality and fat replacement in bakery products continues to be a major area of product research. However, published information on fat function and replacement targeted to baked goods has been scarce. Presently, the medical implications of reduced-fat intake has given fat replacers a lot of publicity, but most of the information about these fat replacers can only be applied to limited types of baked goods (van Gijssel and van der Steen, 1990; Rasper and Kamel, 1989; Harrigan and Breene, 1989).

Fat reduction alone can reduce air incorporation which results in decreased cake volume, uneven texture and tougher eating. Fat reduction in baked goods is often corrected with water addition, which can greatly change the characteristics of a batter or dough. Increased water content can 'water weight' doughs and batters resulting in poor volume, texture, appearance and shelf life of the finished products. Research conducted by van Gijssel and van der Steen (1990) examined the effect of fat reduction alone on the sensory and rheological properties of puff pastry, shortbread and cake. They found that slight reduction in fat content produced significant product changes which sensory evaluation characterized as firm, sticky, granular, soggy and greasy. In addition, results showed that the processing method had a significant effect on the cake properties and could be used to compensate for the undesirable effects of fat reduction.

Many hydrocolloid systems have shown good fat mimetic properties in baked good systems which contain a relatively high finished product moisture content such as cakes. Starches and hydrocolloids can mimic the rheological sensation of fat in the mouth due to the binding and orientation of water in the molecule (Yackel and Cox, 1992). Low dextrose equivalent (DE) maltodextrins derived from potato, tapioca, corn and rice have shown short texture/fat-like qualities when prepared at 20–25% solutions. Acceptable bakery products including layer cakes, muffins, cheese cakes and pound cakes can be prepared with carbohydrate-based fat mimetics without the dryness often characteristic of low-fat products.

Bath et al. (1992) evaluated three commercial starch-based fat replacers: Stellar® (A.E. Staley Manufacturing Company); N-Flate® (National

Starch and Chemical Company); and Rice*Trin 3 Complete® (Zumbro Inc) at 2% addition level (dry form) to replace shortening in white layer cakes. Results showed that the fat replacement cakes displayed higher batter specific gravities with similar batter viscosities. A key finding in this study was the effect fat replacement had on batter temperature during baking. The cake batters containing fat replacers heated quickly and evenly, with little temperature differences between the edge and center of the pan as compared to fat-containing controls. The finished cakes had lower volume and flatter profiles, but with good internal crumb and grain characteristics.

Ang *et al.* (1989) suggested a systems approach to caloric reduction in sweet-type baked goods. Instead of depending on the functionality of only one bulking agent/fat replacer, a combination of different calorie-sparing ingredients was used with desirable effects. This systems approach was illustrated in a reduced-calorie cupcake formulation that used a combination of two powdered celluloses (both insoluble) and polydextrose (which is soluble). A combination of the soluble and insoluble bulking agents worked best in replacing the functional properties of the substituted ingredients. The fat content of the resultant product was reduced by over 50% (Ang *et al.*, 1989). Research conducted by Campbell *et al.* (1992) measured the effect of various calorie-sparing ingredients on the texture of reduced-calorie oatmeal cookies. The replacement of fat with polydextrose, water and emulsifiers had the greatest impact on cookie texture. Fat replacement in sponge cake was limited to 50% using maltodextrin due to adverse effect on density, volume and sensory properties (Bollinger and Freund, 1992).

Murphy *et al.* (1991) used a combination of hydrated polysaccharide hydrocolloids with hydrated insoluble fiber to eliminate or reduce the fat content in baked goods. In addition to fat reduction they found that the hydrated polysaccharide system prevented or controlled moisture migration and maintained softness and shelf life of the baked goods. They postulated that the hydrated gum and fiber functioned as a reservoir of bound moisture which slowly released moisture into the baked good at ambient storage. It was also speculated that the insoluble fiber helped to disrupt the gummy texture that may result from the application of hydrocolloids.

El-Nokali (1991) developed a fat replacement using liquid crystals formed from polysaccharides. He suggests that improved shape, crumb and dough/batter stability are achieved in many baked goods using this fat substitute because the liquid crystals can exist at the interface of a foam, emulsion or dispersion. Reduction in product shrinkage and collapse were also apparent in test samples as compared with controls.

In high or intermediate moisture bakery food systems, emulsifiers are often used in combination with carbohydrate-based fat replacers for optimal ·effects. An example of a fat-reduced cake formula using a combination of hydrocolloid and emulsifier technology is shown in Table 6.9.

Sobczynska and Setser (1991) evaluated combinations of low DE potato maltodextrin with eight different emulsifiers as a replacement for 50 or 100% of the shortening in chocolate layer cake. Emulsifiers included sucrose esters, monoglycerides, succinylated monoglycerides, sorbitan monostearate, polysorbate 60 and sodium stearoyl lactylate. Results of their study showed that most of the fat replacement systems tested produced chocolate cakes comparable to the control. In general, cakes made with sucrose ester had higher volumes while those made with sorbitan monostearate had the lowest volume. In addition, the method of ingredient incorporation had a significant effect on cake volume, with use of hydrated emulsifier and dry maltodextrin providing optimal results.

Lawson and Lin (1992) evaluated the effect of gums and emulsifiers as a dry blend shortening substitute for bakery applications at a use level of 0.01–0.04%. Results showed that the gums/emulsifiers combinations can be used to replace up to 100% of the fat in bakery products such as layer cakes, muffins, devils food cake and cookies.

In some cases, using the right type and/or level of emulsifier(s) can be important. Emulsifiers or blends with a hydrophilic–lipophilic balance (HLB) value above ten will promote uniform distribution of fat into the water system of the cake because these emulsifiers are hydrophilic.

Table 6.9 95% Fat-free cake mix formulation

Ingredient	Total mix (%)	Flour basis (%)
Cake flour	37.14	100.0
Sucrose	28.38	76.4
Krystar 300 fructose	15.57	42.7
Dur-Lo (Van Den Bergh)	4.03	10.8
Non-fat dry milk	3.56	9.6
Ultra-bake NF	2.99	8.0
Dried egg whites	1.79	4.8
Sta-Slim 150 (Staley)	1.67	4.5
Salt	1.41	3.8
Baking soda	0.95	2.6
Stable 9 (Monsanto)	0.51	1.4
Panalite (Monsanto)	0.48	1.3
Creamy vanilla (Universal 464174)	0.48	1.3
Lecithin (Lucas Meyer MCP)	0.32	0.9
Butter vanilla (Fries & Fries)	0.32	0.9
Gatodan 415 (Grindsted)	0.10	0.3

(390 g water to 630 g dry mix)

Source: A.E. Staley Manufacturing Company

However, the use of combinations of emulsifiers with low and high HLB values can generally provide greater emulsion stability (Dartey and Biggs, 1987). Various emulsifiers including mono- and di-glycerides, sodium stearoyl lactylate, sorbitan monostearate and polysorbate 60 have partially or totally replaced fat in reduced-calorie cake products (Kamel and Rasper, 1988; Rasper and Kamel, 1989). The emulsifiers promoted increased aeration and water absorption at high hydration levels which resulted in good quality cakes with low-fat content (3–6% flour weight basis). Emulsifiers also provided tenderization and retention of freshness to baked goods. Rule *et al.* (1982) reduced the caloric content of cake batters and mixes by replacing the fat with a partial glycerol ester emulsifier. The resultant products showed improved texture, volume and grain at a 10 to 25% fat replacement level. Partially digestible mixtures of sucrose fatty acid esters were used to mimic the functionality of shortening and margarine in reduced-calorie baked goods such as cake mixes (Klemann and Finley, 1990).

Many commercial bakeries are utilizing fat replacement technology in their products. For example, General Mills, Pillsbury and Duncan Hines used gums, emulsifiers and fibers to reduce fat content in selected cake mixes. Entenmann's removed shortening and eggs from their fat and cholesterol-free baked goods and replaced them with maltodextrin, emulsifiers and gums. Similar ingredient technology is used by Sara Lee and Campbell Taggart, while Continental Baking has combined portion control and reformulation in its Twinkies® and Hostess Lights® products (Vetter, 1991). In addition, many of the commercial reduced-fat products have higher than normal sugar levels resulting in little if any caloric reduction.

6.3.3 Sugar replacement in baked goods

Sugar provides many functional attributes to baked goods in addition to sweetness. The character of baked goods is greatly dependent on the chemical behavior of sugars. In cookies, high sugar levels combined with low moisture provide the crisp and brittle texture desired in sugar snap cookies. In high moisture systems such as cakes, sugar retards the gelatinization of starch which has a tenderizing effect on cake texture. Sugar also provides humectancy for baked goods which provides moistness, tenderness and a preservative effect.

High-potency sweeteners can be used to replace the sweetness contribution of sugar in reduced-calorie baked goods. In order for them to be effective in bakery systems they must be heat stable. Aspartame is an approved high-potency sweetener but cannot be used in baked goods due to poor heat stability. Alitame exhibits some heat stability, but losses of about 20% have been reported in bakery applications (Freeman, 1989). Acesulfame-K is heat stable but, due to its perceived bitter flavor, only works well when combined with other sweeteners. It is currently being used in some bakery products in Europe. The heat stability of sucralose in baked goods was demonstrated by Barndt and Jackson (1990). They prepared cake, sugar cookies and graham crackers with ^{14}C-sucralose to evaluate a broad cross section of ingredients and thermal processes seen in the baking industry. Results demonstrated that 100% of the radioactive sucralose was recovered from each baked product. Duplicate analysis on each product showed that no loss of sucralose occurred during baking and no breakdown was detected. Furthermore, Hood and Campbell (1990) evaluated the stability of sucralose in cakes, cookies, brownies and graham crackers when exposed to environmental conditions simulating product distribution. After 12 weeks storage at −18, 22 and 35°C no loss of sucralose occurred in any of the products tested.

Reduction of sugar's bulk in baked goods leads to formula imbalance, producing undesirable results. The partial or complete removal of sucrose from cookie dough tends to produce a cookie with a flaky texture typical of biscuits (Finley *et al.*, 1992). In addition, the replacement of sucrose with humectant ingredients tends to produce a soft/chewy texture to the products. The overall changes in sugar-reduced cookies tend to make them less acceptable to consumers in general. Hood and Campbell (1990) showed complete removal of sugar from yellow cake would not provide a one third caloric reduction. In addition, structural failure occurred in the yellow cake when sugar was completely removed (Figure 6.1a). Askar *et al.* (1987) evaluated cakes made to a standard recipe, in which 0–75% of the sucrose was replaced by the equivalent amount of sweetness from fructose, acesulphame-K, aspartame, saccharin, sorbitol or xylitol. Overall, the results showed that partial replacement of sucrose by the other sweeteners studied reduced quality and acceptability. The reduction in quality was small when only 25% of the sucrose was replaced, but this small reduction in sugar provided no meaningful reduction in calories.

The majority of insoluble bulking agents used in reduced-calorie baked goods are mainly dietary fibers derived from grain sources (i.e. corn, wheat, oat, barley), legumes (i.e. pea, lupine, soy), fruits (i.e. apple, pear, date) and stalks and woods (i.e. celluloses). There are currently over 100 commercially available dietary fiber ingredients. In addition, the vast information available on fiber functionality has been useful to bakers in devising successful formulations with fibers (Hegenbart, 1992).

The insolubility of fibers tends to make them non-functional. Often, fibers are dead weight that require the functionality of other ingredients (i.e. protein and starch) to carry them in order to minimize adverse effects on finished product quality (Vetter, 1991). Incorporation of insoluble bulking agents in baked goods often requires special handling or changes in normal unit operations. Dietary fibers tend to absorb large quantities of water which dilute calories, but also result in mixing and dough handling

(b)

(a)

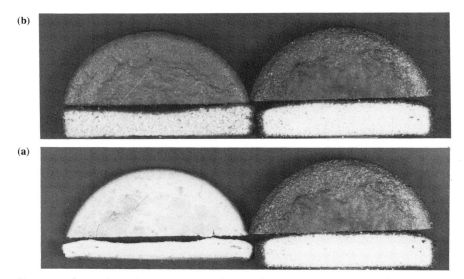

Figure 6.1 Comparison of volume and relative crumb structure in yellow cake formulated as follows: (a) Sugar-free, no bulking agent (left); normal sugar control (right); (b) sugar-free with polydextrose sugar substitute plus increased leavening (left); normal sugar control (right).

problems. The behavior of reduced-calorie products can be affected by the rate of hydration of the fibers. Presoaking fibers prior to use is often necessary to provide the needed functionality.

Insoluble bulking agents have been a key factor in the development of reduced-calorie non-sweet baked goods such as breads and rolls. The high water-holding capacity of insoluble bulking agents is essential because water is a significant ingredient for caloric reduction of these products. Table 6.10 shows a formulation for reduced-calorie bread in which powdered cellulose is used partially to replace a portion of the bread flour. Formulation and processing adjustments are necessary compared to traditional bread formulas since addition of insoluble bulking agents will affect absorption, yeast fermentation, mixing, floor time and cooling (Dubois, 1978).

Recent studies have also shown that some insoluble bulking agents like powdered cellulose can improve the quality of traditional baked goods (Ang et al., 1989; Ang and Miller, 1989). Many calorie-reduced baked goods tend to have structural problems including depressed volumes and crumbly texture due to the effects of reduced-calorie ingredients. Significant volume improvements in yellow cake resulted from incorporation of powdered cellulose at low use levels (Figure 6.2). It has been postulated by Ang and Miller (1991) that stabilization of air bubbles (by cellulose addition) within the cake batter increased cake volume. In addition, textural analysis of the cakes showed texture modification with increased cake firmness.

Table 6.10 Formulation for a reduced-calorie bread

Ingredient	Percent
Sponge	
Bread flour	24.50
Vital wheat gluten (activated)	1.40
Mineral yeast food	0.18
Instant dry yeast	0.52
Water	15.80
Dough	
Bread flour	10.50
Vital wheat gluten (activated)	2.80
Solka-Floc® BW-200FCC	8.40
Granulated sugar	2.40
Carboxymethylcellulose	0.17
Salt	0.95
Monoglycerides (22%, bread softener)	0.18
Ascorbic acid	90 ppm
Water	32.20

Source: American Institute of Baking

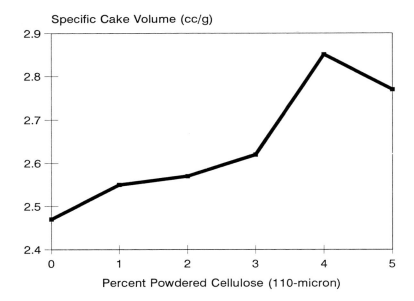

Figure 6.2 Effect of powdered cellulose on the specific volume of yellow layer cake.

There are a variety of soluble bulking agents available to replace the bulk functionality of sugar in baked goods. However, only a few soluble bulking agents have a lower calorie content compared with sugar to make them useful in a reduced-calorie formulation. Polydextrose is perhaps the most recognized and researched low-calorie soluble bulking agent with a reported caloric value of 1 kcal g^{-1}. Isomalt is a disaccharide sugar alcohol with a reported calorie content of 2 kcal g^{-1}. The commercialization of new soluble low-calorie bulking agents is expected to continue with the growth of reduced-calorie products.

Reduced-calorie fruit filling for pie or pastry can be achieved by replacement of sugar using water in combination with a hydrocolloid system. Table 6.11 shows a formulation for a reduced-calorie apple pie in which water, starch and sucralose were substituted for the bulk functionality of sugar. Similar technology can be utilized for development of other fruit varieties and cream/custard pie fillings by selecting the proper hydrocolloid system. Most importantly, existing ingredients and process equipment can be used for this baked goods category.

One of the major effects of using bulking agents/sugar replacements in cookies is the reduction in cookie spread. Replacement of sucrose with

Table 6.11 Apple pie formula

Ingredient	Percentage	
	Control	Reduced-calorie
Filling (75%)		
IQF apples	45.50	60.00
Water	31.30	36.30
Sugar	20.00	0.00
Starch (pregel)	2.80	2.50
Flavors	0.40	0.80
Sucralose (10% solution)		0.40
Total filling	100.00	100.00
Crust (25%)		
Pastry flour	54.01	53.69
Shortening	32.73	26.84
Water		16.11
Whole egg	7.35	
Non-fat dry milk	2.43	
Sugar	1.84	
Dextrose		1.68
Salt	1.24	1.68
Flavor	0.40	
Total crust	100.00	100.00
Calories/100 g in pie	2.10	1.30

Source: McNeil Specialty Products Company, 1991

maltodextrin in cookies tends to produce a brittle rather than crispy texture with a severe reduction in cookie spread (Finley *et al.*, 1992). Campbell *et al.* (1992) reported that use of fiber ingredients including powdered cellulose and oat hull fiber greatly reduced cookie spread in crisp oatmeal cookies when used as a partial flour replacement in combination with reduced-fat levels. The use of a multi-textured cookie dough may help eliminate the textural and spread problems associated with reduced calorie cookies. Finley *et al.* (1992) showed that a dual textured cookie with an outer layer cookie dough containing a glass-forming polysaccharide and humectant sugar surrounding a center dough containing a humectant produced a crisp non-brittle texture.

Rudolph *et al.* (1989) reported on a reduced-calorie oatmeal cookie that used polydextrose to replace up to 60% of the sugar content in combination with sucralose for sweetness. A mixture of corn syrup and fructose was retained in the formula to provide color, flavor and humectancy. The reduced-calorie cookies were similar to controls except for a small reduction in cookie spread. The use of water-soluble polydextrose as a replacement for fats or shortening in cookies was reported by Dartey and Biggs (1987). This approach provided caloric reduction in the cookies by partial fat replacement, thus retaining sugar for its beneficial effect on texture and oven spread.

Combinations of bulking agents are often required to replace the non-sweet functional properties of sugars in baked goods. Frye and Setser (1991) evaluated six bulking agents (sorbitol, a hydrogenated starch hydrolysate mixture, lactitol, isomalt, 18 DE maltodextrin and polydextrose) in reduced-calorie yellow cake totally or partially to replace sucrose. The resultant cakes showed indications of air pockets/puffed crust appearance for all the bulking agents except maltodextrin and polydextrose. They postulated that the lack of air pockets in the maltodextrin and polydextrose samples was due to the increased batter viscosities of these samples. The maltodextrin-containing cakes also had a delicate crumb structure and a thick top crust most likely due to the changes in protein denaturation and/or starch gelatinization. Overall, the reduced-calorie cakes were sensory rated as being between a pound cake and yellow cake.

Dartey and Biggs (1987) developed reduced-calorie cookies by reducing sugar, flour and shortening by using water-soluble polydextrose, and emulsifier and a cellulosic bulking agent. By controlling the pH and leavening during baking, the resultant cookies had a tender open-celled structure with a mouthfeel and appearance of conventional cookies. They also found that use of dry bulking agents in a creaming stage in place of sugar resulted in lump formation and/or gummy texture. Slower addition of the bulking agents reduced this problem, but was not conducive for commercial scale operations. The use of aqueous solutions of polydextroses alleviated incorporation problems.

Research conducted at McNeil Specialty Products Company evaluated the partial replacement of sugar, flour and fat to produce a 35% calorically-reduced chocolate cake (Table 6.12). Sucralose was used at about 500 parts per million in combination with the bulking agent Litesse, starch and a hydrocolloid partially to replace sugar's sweetness and bulk functionality. A 10/12 cocoa was used partially to replace flour, and N-Flate® helped reduce the shortening content. The nutritional profile of the cake is shown in Table 6.13. Sensory evaluation showed the chocolate cake to be comparable to commercial chocolate cake. In addition, the manufacturing process of the reduced-calorie chocolate cake was consistent with current manufacturing processes and equipment. Similarly, Hood and Campbell (1990) used polydextrose to replace sugar bulk in reduced-calorie yellow cakes in combination with an emulsified shortening to replace a portion of the fat (Figure 6.1b). The high-potency sweetener sucralose replaced sweetness lost from sugar replacement. The optimized reduced-calorie yellow cake was comparable to a high quality commercial cake for flavor, texture and overall acceptability.

Singer et al. (1989) showed that a bulking agent comprised of purified cellobiitol could be used in formulating reduced-calorie baked goods to provide texture, moisture retention capability, appearance and density similar to that of sucrose. Baked goods including cookies, cakes, pastries and pies were successfully prepared using a combination of cellobiitol and high-potency sweetener.

Bollinger and Freund (1992) produced a reduced-calorie sponge cake with a combination of 30% sugar substitution by Isomalt, 10% flour/starch

Table 6.12 Product formula for a reduced-calorie chocolate cake

Ingredient	Percentage
Water	43.01
Cake flour	19.03
Whole egg (fresh)	9.51
Shortening	7.23
Fructose	4.76
Polydextrose	4.76
Cocoa	4.28
Wheat starch	2.85
Non-fat dry milk	0.95
Baking powder	2.66
N-Flate	0.38
Salt	0.38
Sucralose (liquid concentrate)	0.20
CMC	0.14
Total	100.00

Source: McNeil Specialty Products Company, 1991

Table 6.13 Nutrition information for a reduced-calorie chocolate cake mix

Description:	Sucralose sweetened chocolate cake mix
Serving size:	3.5 ounces (100 g)
Total caloric reduction of prototype vs. control:	35.80
Calories per serving:	
A. Prototype	220
B. Control	347
C. Approximate cal g^{-1}(finished mix)	2.23
Nutritional content of prototype (grams per serving):	
A. Carbohydrate	36.3
B. Fat	9.91
C. Protein	4.35
D. Sodium	475 mg
Added sweetener profile of product (grams per serving):	
A. Sucrose	—
B. Fructose	5.8
C. Others	—
Caloric contribution (approximate):	
A. From carbohydrate	56%
B. From fat	37%
C. From protein	17%
Market target:	Betty Crocker Chocolate Box cake mix

Source: McNeil Specialty Products Company, 1991

substitution by pea fiber and approximately 40 to 50% fat substitution by maltodextrin. The quality of the cake remained practically unchanged when 20% of the sugar was replaced by Isomalt. Kim (1984) showed that the use of lactitol as the sugar alcohol provides a crispy product when held for several months and protected from moisture.

Dietetic biscuits were produced by Wittig *et al.* (1987) through sucrose replacement with one of the following mixtures of sweeteners: (i) saccharin/sorbitol, 0.25:99.75; (ii) saccharin/sorbitol, 0.35:99.65; (iii) saccharin/fructose, 0.55:99.45 and (iv) sorbitol/fructose, 41.83:58.17. Sensory evaluation of the finished products showed that sweetener mixture (ii) was significantly preferred for color, form, aroma, flavor and texture, while sweetener mixture (iv) was least acceptable. Overall, the products had a 10.9% decease in caloric value as compared to conventional products. In contrast, the same sweetener mixtures were evaluated by Craddock *et al.* (1987) in diabetic almond cookies. Preference tests for the experimental cookies, carried out in a population of 100 adult diabetic patients showed a significant preference (*P* less than 0.01) for cookies sweetened with saccharin/fructose. No significant difference in overall acceptability was detected for any of the sweetener mixtures compared to sucrose controls.

Unlike fat replacement, sugar and calorie reduction of baked goods is not being utilized by many commercial bakeries. Reduced-calorie non-sweet baked products like breads and rolls continue to dominate this category. The majority of commercial reduced-sugar bakery products have been diabetic-related products where sugar is replaced with fructose and/or sugar alcohols. The emergence of new heat stable high-potency sweeteners and suitable low-calorie bulking agents should boost this technology.

6.3.4 Technical issues

With the use of low-calorie food ingredients comes many new challenges. A major concern when developing reduced-calorie baked goods is the effect on shelf life. Many reduced-calorie baked goods exhibit a fresh taste and appearance out of the oven, but they tend to stale rapidly upon storage which provides little to no commercial use. The drying out of these baked goods is more rapid with the reduction of sugars. Since water is normally increased to replace some of the substituted sugar or fat bulk, these products are more susceptible to microbiological spoilage. In addition, the high pH range of most baked goods limits the effectiveness of preservatives to reduce this problem.

Moisture migration is also a major concern in reduced-calorie baked goods. Reduction in fat and sugar increases the water activity of these products making water more readily available for migration. This is especially apparent in baked goods that contain more than one component. For example, a reduced-calorie cake may have a water activity of about 0.9, while the frosting water activity is about 0.75. Within a few days water will migrate from the cake into the frosting to establish equilibrium. The resultant frosting becomes wet and in some cases may even 'melt' off the cake. Similar moisture migration can also occur in snack cake-type products that contain cream fillings and frostings. Moisture migration from the cake into the filling greatly effects the shelf life and quality of the finished products.

The moistness properties that sugars add to baked goods can be easily mimicked by bulking agents, starches, gums and fibers, but the baking properties will change. Without sugars in cakes the starch gelation, protein denaturation and rate of evaporation are all shifted. The surface drying without sugars results in case hardening or crust formation. In addition, the hygroscopicity of many reduced-calorie ingredients tend to pull moisture from the atmosphere which can create clumping and caking problems in bakery mixes. Furthermore, their moisture binding can effect other moisture sensitive ingredients such as leavening systems, flavors and colors.

Addition of solute can make up for lack of sugars. Unfortunately salts, glycols and alcohols will add flavors uncharacteristic of most baked goods. Polydextrose, glycerine and sugar alcohols can produce the effects to some extent with minor flavor changes. In fillings, frostings, icings and other baked goods embellishments, it is easier to approximate the expected textures because they are usually semi-solid or plastic. However, without added solutes the shelf life or freeze–thaw characteristics may not be acceptable.

Calorie reduction in baked goods has a significant impact on freezing properties. Products to be frozen also have defects tied to the sugar solute properties. The removal or reduction of sugar in baked goods tends to elevate freezing points. In addition, product drying (freezer burn) is faster and thaw times are longer from a given temperature below freezing.

Flavor development research is also a challenge for reduced-calorie baked goods. Since taste is a key attribute in determining consumer preference and repurchase intent, formulators need to consider flavor balance early in the development process. Caloric reduction can involve the use of many different ingredient combinations, each of which can alter the flavor release and profile of the finished products. For example, carbohydrate ingredients can complex with lipophilic flavor ingredients which would effect their interaction with the olfactory receptors. Similarly, certain protein-based fat replacers can interact with select classes of flavoring chemical such as aldehydes and ketones. Further investigation of the chemical interaction between food ingredients and flavor chemicals is required to quantify flavor balance in reduced-calorie products (Bennett, 1992).

Regulatory considerations must also be considered when developing reduced-calorie baked goods. The Nutritional Labeling and Education Act of 1990 (NLEA) mandated that the Food and Drug Administration (FDA) publish certain proposed rules by November 8, 1991 covering a broad range of labelling issues. Final rules were to be published by November 8, 1992, with an implementation date of May 8, 1993. Some of the key factors that might impact development and marketing of reduced-calorie baked goods include: serving sizes, analytical methodology to substantiate reduced-fat claims, implied health messages, nutritional and ingredient labeling, and reference foods to be identified when claims are made. Once the regulatory ground rules are established, food technologists and marketers can develop and market reduced-calorie baked goods to help consumers meet their nutritional goals with new and innovative products (Vetter, 1992).

The cost of reduced-calorie bakery products is also important to the success of this product category and the ingredients used in them. Fat replacers, bulking agents and high-potency sweeteners generally cost more than the ingredients they replace. This is due to the high level of technical difficulty in developing these ingredients, and the long and costly time-frame for regulatory approval and commercialization. However, sensitivity to ingredient pricing remains a key issue in the baking industry. Premium pricing of reduced-calorie baked goods is a possible solution to this problem if the product quality is not compromised.

In summary, reduced-calorie baked goods can be formulated with existing low-calorie ingredients, but there are many limitations. Because there is no 'universal' bulking agent and fat replacer, the food formulator must be knowledgeable about the functionality of many ingredients. Often, formulators must select and combine different bulking agents to produce the desired functional characteristics and to achieve the desired caloric reduction. It is common to see a reduced-calorie product contain three or four calorie-reducing ingredients. However, new problems tend to occur as the number of ingredients increases. These changes are primarily tied to eating qualities, but they also have an impact on preparation, storage stability and cost.

6.4 Conclusion

And so the age of 'healthier' sweet baked goods was born in the 1990s. Thus far, most of the new healthy product introductions have been based upon fat and cholesterol reduction or elimination. These healthier products meet the demands of a large segment of the consumer base interested in dieting or just a healthier lifestyle. Since many of these products have been on the market for a year or less, it is too early to know just how successful they will be.

Will these products result in incremental volume to present sweet baked goods sales or cannibalize current product lines? What are the reasons that compel people to go beyond initial purchase and drive repeat purchase intent? Are they value, freshness, quality or taste? Will people be willing to compromise on indulgence in order to limit fat in their diet, or are attributes like value, quality and taste the key to repeat purchase intent? The answer to these questions should become clear over the near term. Long term survival of these healthier products is likely to depend upon the combination of meeting consumer demands for lower fat and calories as well as expectations for taste and quality. Otherwise consumers seem willing to satisfy their need for indulgence with a limited intake of full-calorie sweet baked goods while sparing calories in the remainder of their diet.

The use of new ingredient technology involving gums, stabilizers, emulsifiers and heat stable, high-potency sweeteners such as sucralose will offer the master bakers and food scientists new tools to achieve higher quality caloric reduction. Experience is a great teacher and will lead to a better understanding of how to utilize present and developing ingredient technology in formulation of high quality, nutritionally modified sweet baked goods.

References

Ang, J.F., and Miller, W.B. (1989) Enhancement of cake volume by a new form of powdered cellulose. *Abstract 74th AACC Annual Meeting*, Washington, DC, November 1989.

Ang, J.F. and Miller, W.B. (1991). Multiple functions of powdered cellulose as a food ingredient. *Cereal Foods World*, **36**(7), 558–564.

Ang, J.F., Lee, C.M. and Miller, W.B. (1989) The effect of powdered cellulose on the textural properties of cakes as measured by the Instron. *Abstract 74th AACC Annual Meeting*, Washington, DC, November 1989.

Anon (1991) Pepperidge Wholesome Choice Cookies Meet Fat Guidelines. *Snack Food*, **80**, (10), 34.

Anon (1992a) Dietary fat and cholesterol. *Prepared Foods*, July, 67–70.

Anon (1992b) Newtons Go Fat-Free. *Food & Beverage Marketing*, **11** (3), 40.

Askar, A., Abd-El-Fadeel, M. G., Sadek, M. A., El-Rakaybi, A. M. A. and Mostafa, G. A. (1987) Studies on the production of dietetic cake using sweeteners and sugar substitutes. *Deutsche Lebensmittel-Rundschau*, **83**(12), 389–394.

Barndt, R.L. and Jackson, G. (1990) Stability of sucralose in baked goods. *Food Technol.*, **44**(1), 62–66.

Bath, D.E., Shelke, K. and Hoseney, R.C. (1992) Fat replacers in high-ratio layer cakes. *Cereal Foods World*, **37**(7), 497–501.

Bennett, C.J. (1992) Formulating low-fat foods with good taste. *Cereal Foods World*, **37**(6), 429–432.

Bollinger, H. and Freund, W. (1992) Manufacture of calorie reduced sponge cake. *Food Marketing Technology.*, (**3**) 12–16.

Campbell, L.A., Ketelsen, S.M. and Antenucci, R.N. (1992) Effect of calorie-sparing ingredients on texture of reduced calorie oatmeal cookies. *Abstract 1992 IFT Annual Meeting*, New Orleans, Louisiana, June 1992.

Cauvain, S. (1987) Let them eat cake . . . especially if it's low fat. *Food Flavourings, Ingredients, Packaging and Processing*, **9**(8), 37–39.

Craddock, M., Wittig, E., Araya, V. and Carrasco, E. (1987) Formulation, manufacture, quality evaluations and preference of dietetic cookies for diabetics. *Revista de Agroquimica y Tecnologia de Alimentos*, **27**(3), 417–424.

Dagnoli, J. (1991) Nabisco thinks healthy. *Advertising Age*, **62**(22), 3.

Dartey, C.K. and Biggs, R.H. (1987) Reduced calorie baked goods and methods for producing same. *US Patent*, 4, 668, 519.

Dubois, D.K. (1978) The fiber era: how to modify formulas without problems. *Food Eng.*, (**5**).

El-Nokali, M. (1991) Food products containing reduced calorie, fiber containing fat substitute. *International patent application*, WO 91/18522.

FIND/SVP (1992) The Market for Premium Sweet Baked Goods. FIND/SVP market intelligence report.

Finley, J.W., Verduin, P., Arciszewski, H.E. and Biggs, R.H. (1992) Cookies with reduced sucrose content and dough for production thereof. *US Patent*, 5,080,919.

Freeman, T.M. (1989) Sweetening cakes and cakes mixes with alitame. *Cereal Foods World*, **34**(12), 1013–1015.

Frye, A.M. and Setser, C.S. (1991) Optimizing texture of reduced calorie yellow layer cakes. *Cereal Chem.*, **69**(3), 338–343.

Harrigan, K.A. and Breene, W.M. (1989) Fat substitutes: sucrose esters and Simplesse. *Cereal Foods World*, **34**(3), 261–267.

Hegenbart, S. (1992) In the eye of the storm: using fiber in food products. *Food Product Design*, **2**(1), 19–32.

Hess, J. (1990) Backing talk with action. *Snack Food*, **79**(12), 4.

Hood, L.L. and Campbell, L.A. (1990) Developing reduced calorie bakery products with sucralose. *Cereal Foods World*, **35**(12), 1171–1182.

Kamel, B.S. and Rasper, V.F. (1988). Effects of emulsifiers, sorbitol, polydextrose, and crystalline cellulose on the texture of reduced calorie cakes. *J. Texture Stud.*, **19**(3), 307–320.

Kim, J. C. (1984) Light bakery products for diabetics and method for the preparation of these products. *US Patent*, 4,442,132.

Klemann, L.P. and Finley, J.W. (1990) Edible food composition—comprises a partially digestible mixture of sucrose fatty acid ester(s). *World Patent*, 90-314467/42.

Lawson M. A. and Lin, S. W. (1992) Dry blend shortening substitute for bakery products—comprising xanthan gum, guar gums and emulsifiers, for complete fat replacement in e.g. cakes. *Patent Application*, EP 468552 A2.

Lemieux, R. (1992) Europeans choosing lite lifestyle. *Calorie Control Council News Release*, March.

Liesse, J. and Dagnoli, J. (1990) Appetite grows for 'Light' treats; desserts don't wait for fat substitutes. *Advertising Age*, February, 3.

Malovany, D. and Pacyniak, B. (1991) Projects Lightning and Thunder. *Bakery Production and Marketing*, September, 38–44.

Murphy, G.B., Lang, K.W., Frake, B.N. and Entenmann, W.J. (1991) Process for baked goods and products therefrom. *International patent*, WO 91/19421

Nabors, L.O. (1992) The consumer's view of light foods and beverages. *Cereal Foods World*, June, 425–428.

A.C. Nielsen Scantrack Data (1992). A.C. Nielsen, Nielsen Plaza Northbrook, Illinois 60062–6288.

Rasper, V.F. and Kamel, B.S. (1989) Emulsifier/oil system for reduced calorie cakes. *Oil Chem. Soc.*, **66**(4), 537–542.

Rudolph, M.R., Hood, L.L., Kendall, D.A. and Campbell, L.A. (1989) Application of response surface analysis in the formulation of a reduced calorie oatmeal cookie containing sucralose. Paper presented at Institute of Food Technologists 50th Annual Meeting, Chicago, June 28.

Rule, C.E., Gilmore, C. and Stefanski, E.J. (1982) Low calorie cake batter or mix. *US Patent* 4, 351, 852.

Singer, N.S., Dubois, G.E. and Muller, G.W. (1989) Low calorie bulking agent comprising cellobiitol—to replace bulking and physical properties of sucrose in formulated foods to be sweetened with high potency sweetener. WPI Acc No: 89-178189/24.

Sobczynska, D. and Setser, C.S. (1991) Replacement of shortening by maltodextrin-emulsifier combinations in chocolate layer cakes. *Cereal Foods World*, **36**(12), 983–1054.

van Gijssel, J. and van der Steen, P.J. (1990) Effect of a reduced-fat level on the characteristics of bakery products. *Bakery/Confectionery*, 134–137.

Vetter, J.L. (1991). Calorie and fat modified bakery products. *Am. Inst. Baking Res. Department Tech. Bull.*, **13**(5).

Vetter, J.L. (1992) Impact of new regulations on development and marketing of nutritionally modified bakery foods. *Cereal Foods World*, **37**(6), 433–437.

Wittig, E., Araya, V., Craddock, M., Arteaga, A. and Carrasco, E. (1987) Formulation, preparation and evaluation of rolled and cut biscuits for diabetics. *Archivos Latinoamericanos de Nutricion*, **37**(3), 532–546.

Yackel, W.C. and Cox, C. (1992) Application of starch based fat replacers. *Food Technol.*, **46**(6), 146–148.

7 High-intensity, low-calorie sweeteners
L. HOUGH

7.1 Introduction

The majority of high-intensity sweeteners were discovered by accident rather than by deduction and structural design. In a book entitled 'Serendipity', Roberts (1989) outlines the discoveries, as a result of chance chemical experiment, of saccharin (1) by Fahlberg in 1879, cyclamate (2) by Sveda in 1937 and aspartame (3) by Schlatter in 1965, in each case by the inadvertent tasting of the intense sweetener on their fingers or hands. The early literature of organic chemistry up to the early 1900s, frequently quoted the taste of a new compound as a characteristic, a test that is no longer permitted under the safety at work code of practice, prior to toxicology on the new compound. Important observations include, for example, Emil Fischer's (1890) note that L-glucose was sweet whilst Piutti (1886) discovered that the amino acid D-asparagine was sweet and its L-isomer was not, thereby implicating the intricacies of stereochemistry in the mechanism of sweet sensation.

Approximately fifty very sweet natural products, which are at least 50 times sweeter than sucrose (4), have been discovered in green plants by their taste and qualify as low-calorie sweeteners because of the much smaller quantities required to give equisweetness with sucrose. They have a diversity of chemical structures, apparently unrelated, and include a variety of terpenoids, flavonoids and proteins. A range of monosaccharides, disaccharides, hydrogenated starch hydrolysis products, polydextrose and polyols which are similar in sweetness to sucrose, but less readily metabolised, and are often utilised as bulk sweeteners in dietary and non-cariogenic products. In beverages, it is usual to add such substitutes when high-intensity sweeteners are used in order to give the products body or a similar mouthfeel to sucrose.

The measurement of sweetness is arbitrary since no laboratory instrument is available to carry out the task. In assessing the relative sweetness of a substance, sucrose is invariably used as the standard reference compound, since it has a quick impact, a clean taste and rapid fall off. Sweet substances rarely have the same sweet taste characteristics, nor do they show all of the features associated with the ideal taste and mouthfeel of sucrose. They often vary in the onset time of the sweet sensation, the intensity of sweetness, the quality – sometimes involving bitter, metallic and liquorice flavours – its duration and the aftertastes.

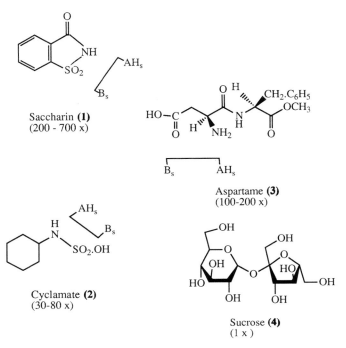

Saccharin (1)
(200 - 700 x)

Aspartame (3)
(100-200 x)

Cyclamate (2)
(30-80 x)

Sucrose (4)
(1 x)

Figure 7.1 Structure of some high-intensity sweeteners and sucrose, their relative sweetness and AH_s/B_s units.

The judgment must be relied upon of a panel of tasters, carefully selected and trained to give their assessments, relative to sucrose, on a weight basis, that is then averaged out to minimise personal variations (Spencer, 1971).

The synthetic sweetener industry commenced sometime towards the end of the last century with the discovery of saccharin (1), initially for use by diabetics and subsequently as a substitute during food shortages in the First World War. However, its safety for the public health has been questioned repeatedly, hence the extensive search for a better, in view of the bitter, metallic aftertaste, and safer high-intensity sweetener, accompanied by a growth in stringent biological testing with a wide range of regulatory procedures for statutory approval of any food additives. Once an intense sweetener has been discovered, this is invariably followed by the chemical synthesis of a wide range of derivatives of related chemical structures, with a view to optimising the sweetness, taste quality and, most importantly, the safety of the product for use in diabetic and dietetic food and drink. The commercial development of a novel sweetener as a food additive requires, of necessity, prolonged and extremely expensive study programmes involving a complex series of pharmacological and toxicological tests. The onus is upon the industry to provide substantial evidence of safety for health of the potential consumers, an area of great concern to the population in the light of past controversies over saccharin and cyclamate (Gunner, 1991). Following the ban on cyclamate (2) in 1970 in the UK and USA, saccharin (1) remained the only high-intensity sweetener to be allowed, but this changed considerably with the 1983 'Sweeteners in Food Regulations', permitting a range of products (Wells, 1989).

The diversity of chemical structures – sugars, amino acids, aromatic compounds and terpenoids – that evoke a sweet taste has stimulated a wide interest in the relationship between chemical structure and sweetness, the stimulatory mechanism and the physiological basis, invariably with a view to designing the ideal non-caloric sweetener. The common feature linking all sweet compounds was recognised as a bifunctional entity, a proton donor (AH_s group) and a proton acceptor (B_s group), in close proximity and separated by only 2.5–4.0 Å (Shallenberger and Acree, 1967), as indicated by the AH_s/B_s designated on structures (1)–(4) in Figure 7.1. There is increasing evidence that the receptor on the taste buds of the tongue is proteinaceous and it appears to be generally accepted that the AH_s/B_s units of the sweet molecule combine with a similar bifunctional system (AH_r/B_r) on the sweet sensitive protein, with the formation of two intramolecular hydrogen bonds which initiate the sweet sensation (Suami and Hough, 1991) (see Figure 7.2).

In order to account for the different degrees of sweetness, a third component of the glucophore was proposed, a hydrophilic unit (X_s), consistent with a stereoselective triad ($AH_s/B_s/X_s$) of binding components (Kier, 1972). The lipophilic group (X_s), sometimes referred to as 'greasy' point, is attracted to a similar site (X_r) on the receptor, probably located on the sidechains of the peptide units, by dispersive forces (van der Waals attraction). The strength of this attraction between X_s and X_r appears to play an important role in determining the intensity of sweetness, as, for illustration, to contrast the low sweetness of the hydrophilic carbohydrates, such as sucrose (4), with the lipophilic, high-intensity sweeteners saccharin, cyclamate and aspartame. Increased hydrophobicity that is built into a molecule will often result in increased sweetness, thus D-tryptophan is 35 times sweeter than its basic unit, glycine. The lack of sweetness in its optical isomer L-tryptophan, has been attributed to a steric requirement, namely that the $AH_s/B_s/X_s$ units should be in a clockwise direction when a chiral sweetener faces the receptor protein (see Figure 7.3). This priority is supported by a combination of stereochemical and taste studies on the chlorosucroses and the isomers of aspartame (3) (Hough and Khan, 1989; Suami and Hough, 1992).

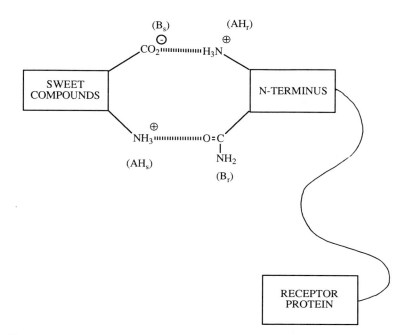

Figure 7.2 Postulated interaction between a sweet amino acid and a protein receptor.

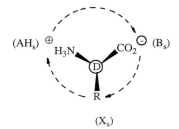

Figure 7.3 Clockwise sequence of $AH_s/B_s/X_s$ units in sweet D-amino acids.

Stereomolecular modelling studies suggest that more than one dispersion bond can be formed to the receptor protein, for instance, in the interactions of the lipophilic methylene groups $(-CH_2-)$ of fructose and sucrose where two or three dispersion bonds $(X_s, X_s', $ and $X_s'')$ are possible to the lipophilic side chains of different amino acid constituents. Another model, deduced from structure–activity relationships, assumes the existence of up to eight sites of recognition. Not all of these groups need to be present in a molecule for sweetness, a minimum of two, but at least four for very high intensity (Tinti and Nofre, 1991).

7.2   Approved artificial sweeteners

7.2.1   Saccharin

Saccharin and its salts (**5**), the sodium salt in particular, have been used as substitutes for sugar for almost a century, despite continual controversy over their safety. Consumption rate increased significantly in North America in the late 1950s from 15 000 kg in 1953 to 2.5 million kg per annum in 1970, due to the rising popularity of dietary food and drink. The easily soluble sodium salt (**5**) is the most commonly used since the parent acid (**1**) is only sparingly soluble in water. Saccharin is non-caloric, not metabolised, and is extensively used in low-calorie drinks because of its potency as a sweetener (>300 times), stability and cheapness (about 2–3% of its sucrose equivalent). The bitter metallic aftertaste of saccharin limits its use singly but this can be overcome by blending with other sweeteners, due to a synergistic effect, with acceptable sweetness characteristics, notably a masking of the aftertaste (Wells, 1989). Unlike sucrose, saccharin has a slow impact and the sweetness gradually builds to a maximum which then persists. The relative sweetness of saccharin declines with increasing concentration and it is also affected by acidity, temperature and type of food and flavour (Wells, 1989).

Following adverse toxicity studies on cyclamate (**2**) in 1970 in the USA, fears of the safety of saccharin led to extensive investigations, but more than twenty reliable studies showed no significant risk of cancer in humans on consumption of large quantities of saccharin. It is now approved almost universally as a food additive, in at least 90 countries. In the UK, the 1983 'Sweetness in Food Regulations' permitted the use of saccharin (Wells, 1989). However, in the USA it contravenes the 'Delaney Clause', because some bladder tumours were found in rats; its use is permitted but must be accompanied by a warning label, 'to give benefit to many for the sake of a very theoretical risk'. An important property of saccharin lies in its role in suppressing dental caries (Grenby, 1991).

The original synthesis of 1879 is still the major industrial process, starting with toluene, at that time a product of the coal tar industry, which

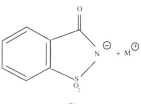

(**5**)

is converted into a mixture of the *ortho-* and *para*-sulphonyl chlorides. After separation of the *ortho*-isomer, it is treated with ammonia to give the sulphonamide which on mild oxidation yields the cyclic amide of *ortho*-sulphobenzoic acid or saccharin.

The activated imino hydrogen, by virtue of the influence of the neighbouring carbonyl and sulphonyl groups, is acidic and hence forms water-soluble salts. At low pH, it slowly hydrolyses to produce non-sweet 2-sulphobenzoic acid and *ortho*-carboxybenzene sulphonamide.

N-Alkyl derivatives of saccharin are tasteless, thus supporting the AH_s/B_s theory, and replacement of the sulphonyl group by the carboxyl group, a phthalimide, also gives a tasteless product. Substitution in the benzene ring modifies the taste, thus halogens and nitro groups introduce more bitterness with a fall off in sweetness. Thiophene analogues, such as (**6**), show a good taste profile, are non-toxic, but are no sweeter than saccharin (Crammer and Ikan, 1977).

7.2.2   Cyclamate

This sweetener, a cyclohexylsulphamic acid, and its calcium and sodium salts (**7**), is 30–40 times sweeter than sucrose and is related in chemical structure to the cyclic sulphamate, saccharin. After its discovery in 1944, its use, primarily in soft drinks, rose to major proportions in the mid 1960s, because of the surprising synergistic effect found with saccharin. A 10:1 mixture of the two doubled in sweetness and together they produced an excellent sweetness by reducing the side tastes of the individual sweeteners. Cyclamate gives clear stable aqueous solutions throughout the pH range and hence in food processing. However, in 1970, its use was banned at the zenith of consumption in the USA and UK following controversial but adverse toxicological investigations. Since then a number of reliable studies have failed to show that cyclamate, or its principal metabolite cyclohexylamine (**8**), is carcinogenic in animals, although it does cause testicular atrophy. Whilst its use is restricted in North America, it is permitted in several European countries, Australia and New Zealand, and has been approved by the Scientific Food Committee of the EC and

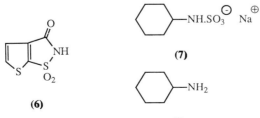

FAO/WHO (Wells, 1989; Grenby, 1991). Because of its relatively low sweetness (30–40 times), cyclamate is more expensive than saccharin (300–600 times), costing about half its equivalent in terms of sucrose sweetness.

The method of synthesis of cyclamate (2) is simple and inexpensive, involving the sulphonylation of cyclohexylamine (8) using chlorosulphonic acid, followed by treatment of the resulting cyclohexylammonium salt with sodium hydroxide and calcium hydroxide to give the desired sodium or calcium salt (7). An alternative synthesis utilises the catalytic reduction of the aromatic sulphamate (Crammer and Ikan, 1977).

Like saccharin, the sweetness of cyclamate disappears when the N–H group is alkylated but N-cyclopentylmethylsulphamate is actually sweeter than cyclamate. The cyclohexane ring is not essential for sweetness since some open chain derivatives, such as the iso-amylsulphamate was 10 times sweeter and the n-butyl derivative 50 times sweeter than sugar. A study of structure activity relationships revealed that to have a sweet taste, the sulphamates must have a —CH—N.R—SO$_3^-$ function (Benson and Spillane, 1976). Apparently a hydrogen substituent must be present on the carbon atom adjacent to the nitrogen atom, this raising the question of where the AH$_s$ function of the AH$_s$/B$_s$ resides?

7.2.3   Acesulfame-K (Von Rymon Lipinski, 1988)

This sweetener was discovered by chance in the 1960s by Clauss and Jenson, at Hoechst AG, whilst investigating a product of reaction between butyne and fluorosulphonyl isocyanate (F.SO$_2$—N=C=O), due to the presence of 5,6-dimethyl-dihydro-oxathiazinone dioxide (10; R$_1$=R$_2$=CH$_3$), at that time a completely novel ring system. The safety dramas of the 1970s stimulated further interest and a range of related structures were synthesised for the evaluation of their toxicities and taste characteristics. Ring substituents at C5 and C6 proved to be beneficial but as expected methylation of the nitrogen cancelled out its sweetness as did

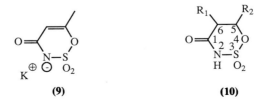

(9)   (10)

small variations within the ring. The most promising compound proved to be the potassium salt of 6-methyl-1,2,3,-oxathiazin-4(3H)-one-2,2-dioxide (**9**), given the generic name of 'Acesulfame potassium salt'. It is about 200 times sweeter than 3% sucrose solutions and costs about 50% of its sucrose equivalent. At higher concentrations, the relative sweetness decreases, hence at 6% solution of sucrose equivalence it is only 100 times sweeter. The quality of sweetness appears to be better than saccharin, it is perceived rapidly but does not fall away as quickly as sucrose. It is not metabolised and has good stability, one of its major advantages, over a range of pH. Synergism is shown with cyclamate and aspartame, but not with saccharin. Interestingly a synergistic effect is also shown with nutritive sweeteners such as fructose and sorbitol.

Acesulfame-K(**9**) is readily synthesised from *tert*-butyl aceto-acetic acid, and the addition product from reaction with fluorosulphonyl isocyanate, when gently heated, gives off CO_2 and isobutene to generate, in high yield, the *N*-fluorosulphonyl aceto-acetic acid amide. The latter cyclises in the presence of base, with the elimination of hydrogen fluoride, to give the oxathiazinone dioxide as its potassium salt, namely acesulfame-K.

Pharmacological and toxicological studies have revealed that acesulfame-K is non-toxic and it has been approved for use in food and drink products in the UK, USA and other countries.

7.2.4   *Aspartame* (Mazur and Ripper, 1979; Homler, 1988)

This dipeptide derivative (**3**) with a sweetness 180–250 times that of sucrose is without doubt the most successful high-intensity sweetener in current use and its impact on the dietary market has been immense, stimulating considerable research studies on related products. After its final approval by the FDA in 1981, worldwide sales of aspartame grew rapidly from $11 million per annum to over $800 million in 1985; sales are predicted to rise to $1.7 billion in this growth market. Under the brand name 'Nutrasweet' it is incorporated into a myriad of low-calorie foods and beverages because its sweetness, combined with taste intensification and flavour enhancement, gives an acceptable taste profile. Shortly, aspartame will come out of

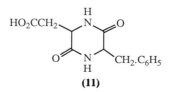

(11)

patent and other companies such as Angus Fine Chemicals in Ireland and VOF of the Netherlands will compete with Nutrasweet.

Despite the fact that the sweetness of various amino acids had been recognised for more than a century, glycine was so renamed because it is sweet, no concerted effort was made to exploit this property, and the dipeptides were ignored. The sweetness of aspartame was discovered by chance in 1965 when Schlatter, at Searle, prepared it as an intermediate during a projected synthesis of a gastrin tetrapeptide for bioassay studies. The original synthesis employed classical methods, by coupling a protected carbobenzyloxy-L-aspartic acid β-benzylester with L-phenylalanine methyl ester, followed by the removal of the protecting groups by catalytic hydrogenation. This scheme was usually followed in the synthesis of at least 1000 related derivatives and analogues. However, this synthesis was far too expensive for commercial purposes and many modifications were introduced to make it cost effective. One alternative approach utilises the knowledge that aspartic acid is an amino-succinic acid yielding a stable anhydride which can be coupled with phenylalanine methyl ester to give a favourable ratio of α/β isomers from which aspartame is readily isolated by solubility differences.

Original anxieties over the safety of aspartame – in the USA it was approved for dry uses in 1974, then withdrawn in 1975, but restored in 1981 – proved groundless, and was later approved for beverages (1983) and many other products. Numerous studies established confidence in the safety of aspartame, and it is now the most popular sweetener in over 75 countries. There are however two drawbacks to the use of aspartame. Those people who suffer from phenylketonuria, a metabolic disease, need to restrict their intake of L-phenylalanine from *all* sources because of their inability to metabolise this α-amino acid; products containing aspartame must therefore carry an appropriate warning! Because aspartame is an ester, under moist conditions it is not stable to heat and undergoes: (a) hydrolysis to the free dipeptide, aspartic acid, phenylalanine and methanol; and (b) cyclodehydration to its diketopiperazine (11), in both cases with loss of sweetness. The extent of degradation is dependent upon moisture content, temperature and pH; the latter is especially important with maximum stability at pH 4.2 but with rapid loss of sweetness outside the range of pH 2.5–5.5. In carbonated beverages, storage for 6 weeks at 20 and 30°C resulted in 11–16% and 28% loss of aspartame, respectively.

Aspartame is metabolised (4 kcal g^{-1}) like any other natural peptide or protein fragment but its caloric value is negligible (0.02 kcal g^{-1}) because such small quantities are consumed. It is only sparingly soluble in water, about 1% w/v at 25°C, and for optimum dissolution heating at 40°C at pH 4 is recommended. However, it can be predissolved in citric acid at room temperature for immediate use. Aspartame is synergistic with a wide range

(12)   (13)

of carbohydrate and intense sweeteners, such as saccharin. It is however much more expensive than saccharin and acesulfame-K, and costs are similar or a little higher, than sucrose on a relative sweetness basis.

The two chiral centres in aspartame (**3**) give four possible diastereoisomers but only the L,L- (**3**) is sweet, the D,D-, D,L-, and L,D- are not, thereby confirming, as with the sweet D-α-amino acids, that the sweetness mechanism is stereospecific when the sweet compound is a chiral molecule. The NH_3^+ and the CO_2^- groups of the L-aspartyl residue are essential for its sweetness and are believed to comprise the AH_s and B_s respectively of the prosthetic glucophore, whilst the hydrophobic fraction X_s is centred on the aromatic group of the phenylalanine unit. Molecular modelling revealed that when aspartame interacts with the *N*-terminal asparaginyl residue of the postulated helical receptor protein, the phenyl group (X_s) can link to the hydrophobic side chain of the fifth amino acid residue (X_r) in the protein helix (Suami and Hough, 1992). None of the other diastereoisomers could form such a three point attachment, thus accounting for their lack of sweetness on steric grounds. The clockwise, three point $AH_s/B_s/X_s$ unit was found only in the L,L-isomer (see Figure 7.4).

Analogue studies have shown the essential sapophoric unit of aspartame to be L-asparagine, hence the presence of the peptide bond appears to be critical for sweetness. The L-aspartyl residue of aspartame can be modified by acetylation of the amino group. Many analogues which are 10 to >100 times sweeter than aspartame have been synthesised. Thus, Fujino *et al.* (1973, 1976) synthesised L-aspartyl-D,L-aminomalonic diester (**12**) and the rigid, bicyclic fenchyl ester (**13**) proved to be an extremely intense sweetener (>25 000 times).

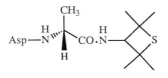

(14)

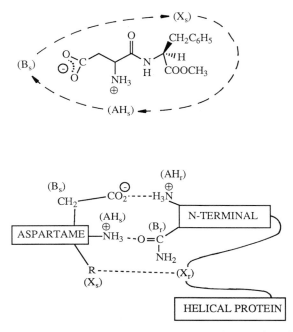

Figure 7.4 $AH_s/B_s/X_s$ groups of aspartame and their postulated interaction with the receptor protein.

Investigation of L-aspartyl-D-alanine amides led Pfizer to develop the 2,2,4,4-tetramethylthietene **(14)**, which is superior to aspartame in solubility, stability and sweetness (2 000 times), and most importantly, does not contain phenylalanine. The product **(14)** has been submitted for approval as a food additive known as 'alitame' (Brennan and Hendrick, 1983), but it is likely to be expensive in view of the more complex synthesis than aspartame. Goodman *et al.* (1987) reversed the usual role of amide structure, a 'retro-inverse peptide' by combining a 1,1-diaminoalkane to a malonic acid derivative leading to a series of very soluble compounds (e.g. **(15)** (900 times sweeter than sucrose), more stable than aspartame, and lacking the undesirable phenylalanine moiety.

7.2.5   *Thaumatins* (Wells, 1989; Higginbotham, 1979; Kim *et al.*, 1991)

This remarkable sweetener is a protein, originally isolated from the fruit of *Thaumatococcus danielli* (Benth.), an African plant named in 1839 after Dr W.F. Danielli, who referred to it as 'Katemfe', the Yorub name. The

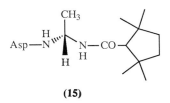

(15)

plant is common throughout the rain forest zone of West Africa, from Sierra Leone to Zaire. Van der Wel and Loewe (1972) isolated two sweet proteins, thaumatin I and II, from homogenates of the arils by ultrafiltration, thus removing low molecular weight materials, followed by separation on ion-exchange chromatography columns. A commercial study by Tate and Lyle showed that greatly increased yields of thaumatin, marketed under the brand name 'Talin', could be obtained by low concentrations of salts, particularly aluminium salts, which also enhanced the colour, stability, purity and sweetness of the product. Yields of total sweet protein quoted are 6 g kg^{-1} of fruit, with a sweetness of 1600–2700 times that of an 8–10% solution of sucrose (Higginbotham, 1977). The product is very soluble in water, stable at pH 2.7–6.0, and apparently can be heated for several hours with little loss in sweetness. However, thaumatin has an unusual taste profile, slow in onset followed by intensification to lingering sweetness with a liquorice-type of aftertaste. A proprietary mixture is available in Japan under the brand name of 'San Sweet T-100' in which thaumatin is combined with alanine, organic acids and filler, thereby doubling the sweetness and reducing both the delay in sweetness and the aftertaste.

An important property of thaumatin lies in its ability to enhance certain flavours and aromas, such as those in peppermint, spearmint, coffee and ginger, where it is likely to find increasing use. As a protein it is metabolised but because of its high sweetness, thaumatin has a low-calorie value per unit of sweetness, less than 0.002 kcal. It is permitted for certain uses in the UK, Australia and Japan but because of its synergism with saccharin, acesulfame-K and stevioside, is often used with one of them in admixture; neither aspartame nor cyclamate shows this effect with thaumatin.

The thaumatin macromolecule has a high overall positive charge causing an association with negatively charged species such as synthetic colours, acidic gums like xanthan, pectin, carboxymethylcellulose, alginate, etc., when loss of sweetness often occurs.

Thaumatins I and II have similar properties, such as amino acid composition, sweetness and molecular weight. Thaumatin I consists of a single chain of 207 amino acid residues with eight disulphide bonds and an X-ray study of its crystal structure has revealed the general features of the protein's backbone (Kim *et al.*, 1991). Also the entire 207 amino acid sequence in thaumatin I has been determined. Heat denaturation of thaumatin or cleavage of the disulphide bridges both lead to loss of sweetness, thus implicating the tertiary structure of the protein in the taste mechanism, probably a highly stereoselective process.

A gene encoding thaumatin, cloned in yeast, was introduced into *Saccharomyces cerevisiae* for thaumatin expression. Several forms of this yeast thaumatin proved to be indistinguishable from the natural plant thaumatin in sweetness intensity and immunoreactivity. Thus, using recombinant DNA technology, variants of thaumatin have been produced by fermentation and several of these proteins display modified taste properties (Weickmann *et al.*, 1989).

Detailed studies on the plant thaumatin have revealed at least five variant proteins in different proportions, and separable from one another on the basis of differing charge characteristics. The two major variants and three minor components (thaumatins a,b and c) are separable by ion-exchange chromatography on different types of resin and using varying solvent systems.

In developing a radioimmune assay (RIA) to determine micro-quantities of thaumatin in food and drink, antibodies to thaumatin were found to be of interest in probing the active site of the sweet proteins. The antibody also recognised other high-intensity sweeteners, including aspartame, leading to the suggestion that the antibody could be used to detect the trigger or active site for the sweet sensation (Hough and Edwardson, 1978; van der Wel and Bel, 1978). The RIA method detects native thaumatin in solutions with as little as 1 ng ml^{-1} of crossreactive protein, one thousand times more sensitive than human taste testing. However, polyclonal and monoclonal antibodies produced against thaumatin are reported to recognise the tertiary structure of the protein but failed to detect aspartame and sucrose (Weickman *et al.*, 1989).

7.2.6   *Steviosides* (Philips, 1987; Crammer and Ikan, 1987)

The extract of the leaves of *Stevia rebaudiana* Bertoni, a variety of the chrysanthemum plant, is a mixture of diterpene glycosides containing as the major components, stevioside (**16**), steviolbioside, rebaudiosides (**17,18**) and dulcoside, which collectively give Stevia 100–300 times the sweetness of sucrose. The plant is indigenous to Paraguay but for economic reasons is now extensively cultivated in South East Asia, Japan and Israel. Attempts to develop a sweetener industry in Paraguay from 1940–1960 met with little success but the Japanese, searching for alternative crops, due to the falling demand for rice, and conscious of the net importation of sucrose into Japan, began trials in 1954, resulting in toxicological evaluation in 1956. Evidence from exhaustive animal studies and use in *homo sapiens*, suggested that it was safe for use, and from 1970 onwards, Stevia has been used in Japan in a wide range of products. However there are contradictory reports on the metabolism *in vivo* of Stevia which would give the mutagenic steviol (**17**).

Since the early products had an unpleasant aftertaste, a menthol or liquorice flavour with some bitterness, much effort was devoted to removing and masking this unwanted property of stevia. Strains have been developed which give a higher proportion of rebaudioside A, a better tasting product than the other constituents. Formulations with cyclodextrin, locust bean gum and L-histidine reduce the aftertaste. Improved versions of stevia have increased sales in Japan from 40 tonnes in 1970 to over 300 tonnes in 1985.

Rebaudioside A (**18**) is more stable, more soluble in water and much sweeter, with a better taste profile, than stevioside (**16**) and can be

O—β—D—Glcp—(2 ← 1) —β—D—Glcp

CH$_3$

H

=CH$_2$

β—D—Glcp—O—C—CH$_3$

H

‖
O

(**16**)

OR$_2$

CH$_3$

H

=CH$_2$

R$_1$O—C—CH$_3$

H

‖
O

(**17**) R$_1$ = R$_2$ = H

(**18**) R$_1$ = β - D - Glcp ; R$_2$ = β - D - Glcp

(2 ← 1) - β - D - Glcp

(3 ← 1) - β - D - Glcp

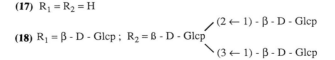

modified by either enzyme transfer of glucose units or chemical treatment further to improve its flavour.

Solutions of stevioside at pH 3–9 when heated at 100°C for 1 hour show little loss in sweetness, and no change at room temperature (22°C) for 5 months, thus demonstrating its high stability. It has been approved for use in Japan since 1972 and in South America, South Korea and China, but has not so far found approval in Europe and North America. It is synergistic with aspartame and acesulfame-K, but not saccharin. On equivalent sweetness basis, its cost is comparable with sucrose.

7.2.7   Neohesperidine dihydrochalcone (NHDC) (Horowitz and Gentili, 1971; Crosby and Wingard, 1979)

Citrus fruits contain bitter flavone glycosides (e.g. (19)), all derivatives of the disaccharide 2-O-α-L-rhamnopyranosyl-β-D-glucopyranose, neohesperidose. In 1963, Horowitz and Gentili found that catalytic hydrogenation of the chalcone form of these flavanone glycosides gave dihydrochalcone neohesperidosides, several of which were, surprisingly, intensely sweet. Numerous dihydrochalcone derivatives were then synthesised for taste and toxicity trials, from which NHDC (20) emerged as a promising high-intensity sweetener, low in caloric value, but unfortunately with aftertaste problems. Thus, neohesperidin (19) undergoes ring opening with sodium hydroxide to give, after catalytic hydrogenation, the sweet dihydrochalcone NHDC. Neohesperidin (19) is the major flavanoid constituent of seville oranges (Citrus aurantium). The dihydrochalcones are colourless, crystalline solids which on tasting show a slow build up of sweetness, rising to 250 times that of sucrose, but more persistent, and with a liquorice/menthol aftertaste but lacking bitterness. An improved taste profile can be obtained by admixture with D-gluconic acid, or its lactone, which reduces the slow onset.

NHDC is only sparingly soluble in water (0.05 g/100 ml), stable at pH 2.5–3.5 and shows a sweetness synergism with saccharin. It is approved for use in Belgium and Argentina, but not in the UK or North America. However, the 'Scientific Committee for Food' in the EC have recommended a daily intake of 5 mg kg^{-1} body weight. NHDC is not absorbed in the small intestine but later does undergo glycosidic cleavage releasing the aglycone.

The essential elements for the sweet taste and potency of the NDHCs are centred around the aromatic nucleus, not the carbohydrate, since 4-O-(carboxy-alkyl) (21) and 4-O-(sulphoalkyl) (22) derivatives are intensely sweet (500 times) and show good solubility in water (Dubois et al., 1977, 1981). However, the overall taste characteristics remain in favour of NHDC.

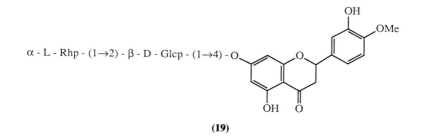

α - L - Rhp - (1→2) - β - D - Glcp - (1→4) - O

(19)

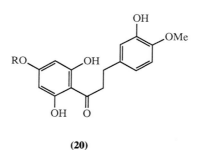

(20)

7.2.8 *Glycyrrhizin* (Crosby and Wingard, 1979; Crammer and Ikan, 1977)

Although it is not generally recognised as a high-intensity sweetener, this terpenoid glycoside (**23**) is 50 times sweeter than sucrose, and finds low-level use in a wide number of products in the flavour, food and pharmaceutical industries because of its unique sweet liquorice flavour. Glycyrrhizin (**23**) is the principle constituent of liquorice root (*Glycyrrhizia glabra* L.) and is composed of a triterpenoid hydroxy-acid, termed glycyrrhetic acid, linked to a (β-1→2) disaccharide, containing two molecules of D-glucuronic acid. It comprises about 6–14% of the dry weight of the roots. The strong liquorice flavour of glycyrrhizin limits its use as a pure sweetener.

Glycyrrhizin is usually isolated from the root extracts, by first removing gums and starches by alcohol precipitation, secondly by addition of sulphuric acid to give a crude, dark precipitated product, which can then be dissolved in aqueous ammonia and crystallised from 95% alcohol. After several crystallisations a pure colourless mono-ammonia glycyrrhetinate is obtained. Acid hydrolysis of glycyrrhizin cleaves the glycosidic bond to give D-glucuronic acid and glycyrrhizic

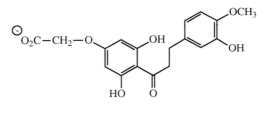

(21)

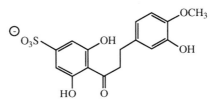

(22)

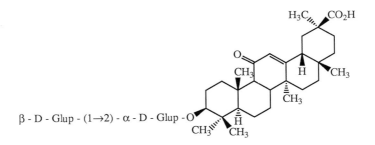

(23)

acid which, incidentally, is tasteless, thereby implicating the disaccharide in the sweetness mechanism.

Glycyrrhizin shows anti-inflammatory activity, similar to that of the glucocorticoids, hence it should be used in moderate amounts as a flavour sweetener because of its pharmacological action (Sela and Steinberg, 1989).

7.2.9 Sucralose (Hough and Khan, 1989; Jenner, 1990)

The considerable enhancement of the sweetness of sucrose, by over 350 times, observed when four of its eight hydroxyls, at or close to the terminal methylene groups, were replaced by chloro groups to give 4,6,1′,6′-tetradeoxy-4,6,1′,6′-tetrachloro*galacto*sucrose (**24**), led to collaborative studies by groups at Queen Elizabeth College (London) and Tate and Lyle (Reading) for the synthesis of a wide range of deoxy-halogeno-derivatives for taste and pharmacological evaluation (Hough *et al.*, 1977). These studies focused attention on 'sucralose', 4,1′,6′-trideoxy-4,1′,6′-trichloro-*galacto*sucrose, a crystalline product over 600 times sweeter than its parent sucrose, which was selected for commercial development by Tate and Lyle (UK) and Johnson and Johnson (USA). In 1991, sucralose was approved in Canada for use in a wide range of food and beverage categories, under the brand name of 'Splenda', as a high-intensity zero-calorie sweetener, and has been submitted for approval in many other countries, including the UK and USA. Sucralose is safe for human consumption having undergone over a hundred rigorous tests, with the advantage that it is extremely stable in finished products and the manufacturing food processes, and is not metabolised on consumption. It has an excellent taste profile, resembling sugar, is very soluble in aqueous systems (28 g/100 ml at 20°C), with no unpleasant aftertaste. On storage for over one year at room temperature at pH values found in most foods and beverages, there was no significant loss of sweetness, and furthermore it does not present any problems by interaction with other food ingredients. The products of hydrolysis with acid are 4-chloro-deoxy-D-galactose and 1,6-dideoxy-1,6-dichloro-D-fructose, whilst base leads to the intramolecular anhydride, 1′,4-dichloro-1′,4-di-deoxy-3′,6′-anhydrogalactosucrose; none of these by-products is sweet.

The original synthesis of sucralose (**25**) from sucrose involved six steps:

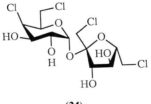

(**24**)

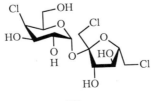

(**25**)

trilylation, peracetylation, detritylation, migration of the 4-acetate group to C-6 followed by chlorination and deacetylation. An improved, especially more economic, synthesis of sucralose has been described by Khan and Mufti (1982), which utilises the concept of selective protection of the 6-hydroxyl group in sucrose with an ester function and then selective chlorination at 4-,1'- and 6'- positions followed by removal of the ester group. Mentech (1989) has achieved the synthesis of the key intermediate, sucrose 6-ester, in 80% yield with benzoic acid and the Mitsunobu reagents, di-isopropylazodicarboxylate in dimethylformamide.

The size of the 6-substituent in sucrose is critical for sweetness, since small groups such as 6-deoxysucrose and 6-O-methylsucrose are sweet, whereas the sucrose 6-acetate is only slightly sweet, and the sucrose 6-benzoate is not sweet. Centres of sweetness enhancement in the sucrose molecule were found at C4 (axial), C1' and C6' when lipophilic halogen substituents were introduced at these positions. Thus replacement of each hydroxyl groups at these centres by halogen resulted in enhanced sweetness, and the effect was synergistic, sweetness increasing to 20 times in the 1'-chloride, to 120 times in the 4,1'-dichloride, and to 600 times in the 4,1',6'-trichloride (25); significantly the 4,1',4',6'-tetrachloride (26) was 2200 times sweeter than sucrose. The special importance of the 4'-position was revealed, when the 4'-bromide (27) and the 4'-iodide (28) were found to be 3000 and 5000 times as sweet as sucrose, respectively.

The AH_s/B_s unit of the sweet halogeno-sucrose has been assigned to the 3'-hydroxyl and 2-hydroxyl, respectively (29), since modifications of either hydroxyl groups resulted in the loss of sweetness. The $AH_s/B_s/X_s$ glucophores in sucralose are in clockwise arrangements. Thus the side chains of the taste bud protein are probably involved in hydrophobic interaction with the regions of lipophilicity in the sucralose molecule which reside largely on the fructosyl unit but extending to the 4-position of the glucopyranosyl unit (29), and probably involving three dispersion bonds centred on C6, C1' and C6' (Suami and Hough, 1992).

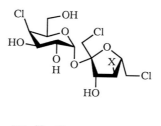

(26) X = Cl
(27) X = Br
(28) X = I

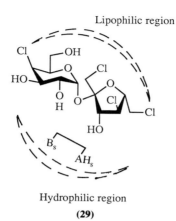

Hydrophilic region

(29)

7.3 High-intensity sweeteners under development

7.3.1 *Monellin* (Ariyoshi *et al.*, 1991; Kim *et al.*, 1991)

This sweetener is a protein isolated by extraction of the berries of a West African plant, *Dioscoreophyllum cumminsi*, and shows similar taste profile to thaumatin. However, these two sweeteners have no obvious similarities in structure, such as amino acid sequences and three-dimensional backbone. Interest in monellin was stimulated by Inglett and May (1968) who named the fruit 'serendipity berries'; extraction procedures yielded 3–5 g of protein per kg of fruit, with 1500–2000 times the sweetness of a 7% sucrose solution on a weight-for-weight basis. After prior tasting of a 0.6% solution of sucrose, the subsequent sweetness intensity of monellin apparently rises significantly, to the enhanced value of 8000 times. The intact macromolecule in its natural tertiary conformation appears to be essential for sweetness. Thus heat denaturation of the protein or partial enzyme hydrolysis causes loss of sweetness.

Monellin has two separate non-covalently bonded sub units, A and B, containing 44 and 50 amino acid residues respectively, but neither sub unit is sweet, one requiring the other, and on remixing they gradually generate sweetness but to only 12% of the original value.

Monellin has been redesigned by genetic engineering to increase its thermal stability and to facilitate its ability to renature. Several of these genetically modified monellins, with only single chains and different linker sequences, are sweet.

7.3.2   Miraculin (Higginbotham, 1979)

The shrub *Richardella dulcifico* Bachni, indigenous to tropical West Africa, yields the 'miracle fruit' which has no particular taste characteristics on its own, but when administered with a sour or acid tasting product, such as vinegar or lemon juice, remarkably produces a persistent sweet taste. Bitter or salty products do not show this transformation with miraculin. The active product in miraculin is a glycoprotein, but this macromolcule is difficult to isolate and purify, and it is unstable, being thermolabile and inactivated below pH 3.0.

Miraculin has a molecular weight of 42000 ± 3000 and is composed of 370 amino acids units in addition to carbohydrate components. Whilst miraculin is unlikely to find approval as a sweetener, it is a fascinating tool or probe for physiological research into the mechanism of sweetness sensation.

7.3.3   Urea and thiourea derivatives: suosan and super aspartame

Dulcin (*p*-ethoxyphenyl urea, **30**) was discovered by Berlinblau in 1884 to have 200 times the sweetness of sucrose, but unfortunately it is toxic. Petersen and Müller (1947) investigated a range of related derivatives, discovering the interesting molecule termed suosan [*N*-(*p*-nitrophenyl)-*N*-(β-carboxyethyl) urea, **31**] which was 350 times sweeter than sucrose, and significantly, the thiourea analogue (**32**) was even sweeter (600 times) (Crosby and Wingard, 1979).

Nofre and Tinti (1991) designed several highly potent sweeteners by combining elements of the suosan family of sweeteners, thiocyanato-suosan for example, with those of aspartame. Amongst these hybrids, a

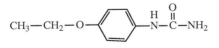

(30)

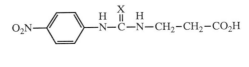

(31) X = O
(32) X = S

'thio-super aspartame' (**33**) with a sweetness of up to 40 000 times that of sucrose was obtained, again the thioureido derivative was more potent than its oxygen analogue, 'super aspartame' (**34**) (14 000 times).

7.3.4 Guanidino derivatives: sucrononic acid (Tinti and Nofre, 1991)

Structure activity relationships in the histamine-H_1 and -H_2 receptor antagonists suggested that the *N*-cyano-guanidine group functions as an effective bioisosteric substitute for the thioureido group. Using this chemical device they developed a new family of potent sweeteners (**35**) based on guanidine. One particular compound (**36**) termed 'sucrononic acid' is the most powerful synthetic sweetener so far encountered (>200 000 times); thus 1 pound weight of sucrononic acid is equivalent to 100 tonnes of sugar. Molecular modelling of sucrononic acid with a helical proteinaceous receptor recorded an excellent fit between the stimulus and the receptor molecules with eight possible binding sites, AH_s (NH_3^+), B_s (COO^-) to the *N*-terminus and lipophilic and dipole interactions with the 5th, 8th and 9th amino acid side chains. This model is an important template for future synthetic studies (Suami and Hough, 1992).

7.3.5 Alitame (Glowaky *et al.*, 1991)

A highly potent dipeptide sweetener was designed from structure–activity relationship studies at Pfizer Central Research, utilising a terminal amide group instead of the methyl ester constituent of aspartame (**3**) in order to improve the hydrolytic stability. The incorporation of D-alanine as the second amino acid, in place of L-phenylalanine, gave the optimum sweetness of the various amino acids tested; significantly the L-amino acids tested were not sweet. A wide range of amines were then incorporated into the L-aspartyl-D-alanyl amide structure. Increased steric and lipophilic bulk on small rings led to high sweetness potencies, with another sulphur

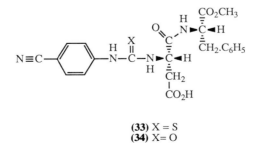

(**33**) X = S
(**34**) X = O

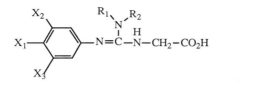

$$X_1 = CN \atop X_2 = X_3 = H \Big\}$$ $$X_1 = H \atop X_2 = X_3 = Cl \Big\}$$

(35)

$R_1 = H$ or CH_3
$R_2 = $ Hydroxy proline

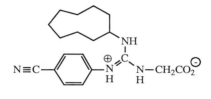

(36)

derivative **(14)**, derived from 2,2,4,4-tetramethyl-3-aminothietane **(37)** proving to be highly sweet (2000 times) and suitable for development in the knowledge that it showed good taste qualities.

Alitame is a crystalline solid, soluble in water (13% w/v at pH 5.6) and significantly more stable than aspartame. A food additive petition was submitted to the US FDA in 1986 and approval is awaited.

7.3.6 *Monatin*

This indolyl-glutamic acid **(38)** was isolated from the ground roots of *Schlerochiton ilicifolius*, a shrub that is native to the North West Transvaal,

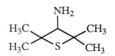

(37)

South Africa. The basic product is isolated by aqueous extraction of the roots, transferred to a cationic exchange resin (H^+ form), then eluted with ammonium hydroxide and finally purified by gel filtration. The product is 1100–1200 times sweeter than sugar but is reported to have a slight liquorice aftertaste (Van Wyk and Ackerman, 1988; Vleggar *et al.*, 1992).

Monatin was identified as (2*S*,4*S*)-4-hydroxy-4-(3-indolylmethyl) glutamic acid (**38**) by nuclear magnetic resonance spectroscopy.

7.4 Conclusions

Regulatory issues on the use of low-calorie sweeteners, initiated by their approval for use as additives in food and beverages, limited or otherwise, vary widely from one country to another. The EC commitment for a single market for food requires the enactment of a sweetener Directive for 1993–1994. This directive will contain a list of high-intensity low-calorie sweeteners with a specified maximum dose for each particular drink, constructed from safety data supplied by their 'Scientific Committee for Food'. The suggested list (see Table 7.1) gives the suggested acceptable daily intake, but these proposals are likely to be controversial with the great diversity of food and opinions across the community. Some of the sweetener levels proposed are insufficient to give the required sweetness to a particular product. Naturally, no manufacturer is going to add more sweetener than is required and it is difficult to see how an individual's daily intake can be controlled.

There would appear to be a good argument for an educative approach, thereby self-limiting, based on suitable labelling of the products, with a specification of the recommended daily intake of the particular sweetener(s) used in the product. The majority of products will undoubtedly utilise a combination of sweeteners in order to take full advantage of sweetness synergism, cost and the quality of the taste profile in a particular food or beverage.

Manufacturers have to be aware of a considerable body of regulatory requirements that relate to both labelling and the use of claims for products

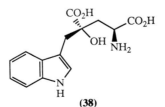

(**38**)

Table 7.1 Maximum quantity of a high-intensity sweetener that can be used in a food or drink in mg l^{-1}or in mg kg^{-1}

Product[*]	Saccharin	Aspartame	Acesulfame-K	Cyclamate	NHDC
Soft drink	80–100	600	350	400	30–50
Beer	80	600	350	—	10
Snacks	100	500	350	—	—
Desserts	100	1,000	350	250	50
Confectionery	300–800	1–2000	500–1000	500	100–150
Chewing gum	1200	5500	2000	1500	400
Ice cream	100	800	800	250	50
Jams, jellies, etc.	200	1000	1000	1000	50
Canned fruit and vegetables	200	1000	350	1000	50

[*]Thaumatin is permitted in confectionery only, at a level of 50

containing novel sweeteners. Health claims on the packaging of foods and beverages, improved taste, better flavour, etc., undoubtedly improve sales of these products, hence the discovery and development of food additives with novel properties will continue to be a priority for the food and drink industry, despite the enormous development costs that can be involved. The world demand for high-intensity sweeteners appears to be insatiable, judging from the ever increasing sales of these products.

A detailed knowledge of the mechanism of action of sweeteners is lacking and is restricted in the main to the relationship of a chemical structure and its conformation to sweetness intensity. The recognition of AH_s/B_s systems in sweet molecules and the associated lipophilic centres will play a key role in future developments. Some insight into the trigger mechanism is emerging from stereoselectivity of the sweet chiral molecules. The high intensity of sucrononic acid and the excellent fit in molecular modelling with a helical receptor protein reveals an important criterion for future studies. The interaction of sweeteners with the taste bud protein and the consequent physiological and neurological stimulatory processes will continue to stimulate scientific enquiry into the intricacies of this most basic of the human instincts.

Acknowledegment

The author is grateful to Professor Benito Casu for providing facilities at the Ronzoni Institute, Milan, Italy, during the compilation of this article.

References

Ariyoshi, Y., Kohmura, M., Hasegawa, Y., Ota, M. and Nio, N. (1991) Sweet peptides and proteins. In: *Sweeteners: Discovery, Molecular Design and Chemo-reception* (eds E.

Wallers, F.T. Orthoefer and G.E. Dubois). ACS Symposium Series 450, ACS, Washington DC pp. 41–60.

Benson, G.A. and Spillane, W.J. (1976) *J. Med. Chem.*, **19**, 869.

Brennan, T.M. and Hendrick, M.E. (1983) *US Patents*, 4,411, 925 and 4,399,163.

Crammer, B. and Ikan, R. (1977) *Chem. Soc. Rev.*, **6**, 431–565.

Crammer, B. and Ikan, R. (1987) Progress in the chemistry and properties of rebaudiosides. In: *Developments in Sweeteners—3*, (ed. T.H. Grenby). Elsevier Applied Science, London and New York, pp. 45–64.

Crosby, G.A. and Wingard R.E. Jr., (1979) A survey of less common sweeteners. In: *Developments in Sweeteners—1* (eds C.A.M. Hough, K.J. Parker and A.J. Vlitos). Applied Science, London, pp. 135–164.

Dubois, G.E., Crosby, G.A., Stephenson, R.A. and Wingard, R.E., Jr. (1977) *J. Agric. Food Chem.*, **25**, 763.

Dubois, G.E., Grosby, G.A. and Stephenson, R.A. (1981) *J. Med. Chem.*, **24**, 408.

Fischer, E. (1890) *Ber.*, **23**, 2611.

Fujino, M., Wakimasu, M., Tanaka, K., Aoki, H. and Nakijima, N. (1973) *Naturwiss.*, **60**, 351.

Glowaky, R.C., Hendrick, M.E., Smiles, R.E. and Torres, A. (1991) Development and uses of alitame. In: *Sweeteners: Discovery, Molecular Design and Chemo-reception* (eds D.E. Walters, F.T. Orthoefer and G.E. Dubois). ACS Symposium Series 450, ACS, Washington DC, pp. 57–67.

Goodman, M., Coddington, J., Mierke, D.F. and Fuller, W.D. (1987) *J. Am. Chem. Soc.*, **109**, 4712–4714.

Grenby, T.H. (1991) *Chemistry in Britain*, 342.

Gunner, S.W. (1991) Novel sweeteners: regulatory issues and implications. In: *Sweeteners: Discovery, Molecular Design and Chemo-reception* (eds D.E. Walters, F.T. Orthoefer and G.E. Dubois). ACS Symposium Series 450, ACS, Washington DC, pp. 302–312.

Higginbotham, J.D. (1977) *US Patent*, 4,011, 206.

Higginbotham, J.D. (1979) Protein sweeteners. In: *Developments in Sweeteners—1* (eds C.A.M. Hough, K.J. Parker and A.J. Vlitos) Applied Science, London, pp. 87–123.

Homler, B. (1988). Nutrasweet brand sweetener: A look beyond the taste. In: *Low-calorie Products*, (eds G.G. Birch and M.G. Lindley). Elsevier Applied Science, London and New York, pp. 113–125.

Horowitz, R.M. and Gentili, B. (1971) Dihydrochalcone sweeteners. In: *Sweetness and Sweeteners* (eds G.G. Birch, L.F. Green and G.B. Coulson). Applied Science, London, pp. 69–80.

Hough, C.A.M. and Edwardson, J.A. (1978) *Nature*, **271**, 381.

Hough, L. and Khan, R. (1989) Enhancement of the sweetness of sucrose by conversion into chloro-deoxy derivatives. In: *Progress in Sweeteners* (ed T.H. Grenby). Elsevier Applied Science, London and New York, pp. 97–120.

Hough, L., Phadnis, S.P., Khan, R. and Jenner, M.R. (1977) *UK Patent*, 1,543,167; *Chem. Abstr.*, **87**, 202019 *v*.

Inglett, G.E. and May, J.F. (1968) *Econ. Bot.*, **22**, 326.

Jenner, M.R. (1990) Sucralose. In: *Sweeteners: Discovery, Molecular Design and Chemo-reception* (eds D.E. Walters, F.T. Orthoefer and D.E. Dubois). ACS Symposium Series 450, ACS, Washington DC, pp. 68–87.

Khan, R. and Mufti, K.S. (1982) *UK Patent*, 2,079,749.

Kier, B.K. (1972) *J. Pharm. Sci.*, **61**, 1394.

Kim, S.H., Kang, C-H. and Cho, J-M. (1991) Sweet proteins. In: *Sweeteners: Discovery, Molecular Design and Chemo-reception* (eds E. Walters, F.T. Orthoefer and D.E. Dubois). ACS Symposium Series 450, ACS, Washington DC, 28–40.

Mazur, R.H. and Ripper, A. (1979) Peptide-based sweeteners. In: *Developments in Sweeteners—1* (eds C.A.M. Hough, K.J. Parker and A.J. Vlitos) Applied Science, London, pp. 125–134.

Mentech, J. (1981) *Eur. Patent*, 0,356,304.

Nofre, C. and Tinti, J-M. (1991) *Eur. Patent Appl.*, 0 107 597.

Petersen, S. and Müller E. (1947) *Chem. Ber.*, **81**, 31.

Philips, K.C. (1987) Stevia: steps in developing a new sweetener. In: *Developments in*

Sweeteners—3 (ed. T.H. Grenby). Elsevier Applied Science, London and New York, pp. 1–44.

Piutti, A. (1886) *C.R. Acad. Sci. Paris*, **103**, 134–137.

Roberts, R.M. (1989). *Serendipity: Accidental Discoveries in Science*. John Wiley, New York, pp. 150–154.

Sela, M.N. and Steinberg, D. (1989) Glycyrrhizin: the basic facts plus medical and dental benefits. In: *Progress in Sweeteners* (ed. T.H. Grenby). Elsevier Applied Science, London and New York, pp. 71–96.

Shallenberger, R.S. and Acree, T.E. (1967) *Nature*, **211**, 75.

Spencer, H.W. (1971) Taste panels and the measurement of sweetness. In: *Sweetness and Sweeteners* (eds G.G. Birch, L.F. Green and C.B. Coulson). Applied Science Publishers, London, pp. 112–129.

Suami, T. and Hough, L. (1991) *J. Carbohydrate Chem.*, **10** (5), 851

Suami, T. and Hough, L. (1992) *J. Carbohydrate Chem.*, **11** (8), 953–967.

Tinti, J-M. and Nofre, C. (1991) Design of sweeteners. In: *Sweeteners: Discovery, Molecular Design and Chemo-reception* (eds D.E. Walters, F.T. Orthoefer and G.E. Dubois). ACS Symposium Series 450, ACS, Washington DC, pp. 88–99.

Van der Wel, H. and Bel, W.J. (1978) *Chem. Senses and Flavour*, **3**, 99.

Van der Wel, H. and Loewe, K. (1972) *Eur. J. Biochem*, **31**, 221.

Van Wyk, P.J. and Ackerman, L.G.J. (1988) *US Patent*, 4,975,298A; (1990) *Chem. Abstr.*, **112**, 177264 *w*.

Verlander, M.S., Fuller, W.D. and Goodman, M. (1986) *US Patent* 451,345; *J. Amer. Chem. Soc.*, **107**, 5821.

Vleggaar, R., Ackerman, L.G.J. and Steyn, P.S. (1992) *J. Chem. Soc., Perkin Trans.*, 3095–3098.

Von Rymon Lipinsky, G.W. (1988) Acesulfame-K. In: *Low-calorie Products* (eds G.G. Birch and M.G. Lindley). Elsevier Applied Science, London and New York, pp. 101–112.

Weickmann, J.L., Lee, J-H., Blair, L.C., Ghosh-Dastidar, P. and Koduri, R. (1989) Exploitation of genetic engineering to produce novel protein sweeteners. In: *Progress in Sweeteners* (ed. T.H. Grenby). Elsevier Applied Science, London and New York, pp. 47–69.

Wells, A.G. (1989) The use of intense sweeteners in soft drinks. In: *Progress in Sweeteners* (ed. T.H. Grenby). Elsevier Applied Science, London and New York, p. 169.

8 Low-calorie soft drinks

M. MATHLOUTHI and C. BRESSAN

8.1 Introduction

The low-calorie soft drinks discussed in this chapter have recently been reviewed (Wells, 1989; Houghton, 1988), but as the subject is continuously changing, a fresh view is justified. The advent of aspartame has led to the availability of good quality soft drinks which has stimulated consumers' demand for tasty food and drinks. As a result there has been interest in low-calorie sweeteners both from scientific and commercial points of view (Houghton, 1988; Wells, 1989). From technical considerations the mechanistic understanding of sweet taste chemoreception incites scientists both from academic and industrial sources. Hundreds of new synthetic sweeteners have been synthesised and evaluated for their sweetness. From the economic point of view it should be stressed that intense sweeteners, although only representing a small tonnage, are likely to increase in market size to around $2.4 billion in the mid 1990s (Wilkinson, 1988). The beverage market is the main user of high-potency sweeteners. After a fast growth between 1983 and 1990, the market for the low-calorie soft drinks has recently shown signs of slowing down. The increase in sales in the USA in the 1980s was in the two-digit region. However, recently diet sales showed a 9.2 and 2.6% growth in 1990 and 1991, respectively (Maxwell Jr., 1992). There are several reasons for this sluggish growth, the most important of these being the saturation of the adult market, the shrinking teenage market, higher prices, a change in pack sizes and above all, the recession. The market boom of the eighties neatly corresponds to the advent of aspartame on the one hand and to the evolution of the safety regulations on the other, especially in Europe. Although growth is now slower, there are opportunities for new products in the market of low-calorie soft drinks which hold 29.8% of the total soft drink market in the USA (Maxwell Jr., 1992), around 26% in the UK and 10% in France (Grimanelli, 1992). A conservative projection for the year 2000 gives an annual growth of 2% for the whole soft drink market (Anon, 1992a), and the most optimistic forecasts estimate the increase at around 5% in the USA and 15% in Europe for the low-calorie soft drinks.

It is noteworthy that sugar (sucrose) has been almost completely removed from soft drinks in the USA. However, this is less likely to happen in Europe especially in France and Italy, because of the strong sugar lobby. The American attitude towards diet is different from the European way, and the lobbying of the sugar industry in Europe is more vociferous. Moreover, the changing mood of the consumer is now much more oriented towards 'healthier' foods than just low-calorie products. Recently, nutritional arguments and media advertisements have stressed quality foods and the well being associated with a healthy diet rather than weight or calories. This is the reason why carbohydrates are increasingly used in conjunction with intense sweeteners, and the artificial sweeteners are chosen for their quality of taste and closeness to sucrose rather than intensity of sweetness. The functional properties of sucrose other than sweetness, required in the formulation of diet beverages, are achieved by the use of low-calorie bulking ingredients. The industry appreciates that there can be no compromise on the consumers' preference for quality and taste in soft drinks.

8.2   Market and technical needs

8.2.1   Consumers and statistics

The consumption of soft drinks has enjoyed strong growth in the USA and throughout Europe in the past years (see Table 8.1).

This trend originates from a change in lifestyle internationally. Americans continue to like 'something nice to drink' for themselves and their families (Sfiligoj, 1992). A recent survey conducted in the UK, France and Germany revealed that 64% of adults (age 18 and older) consume some low-fat or low-calorie foods (Anon, 1992b). The most popular low-calorie products are 'light' (or 'lite') soft drinks which are consumed by 28% of the total population in UK, 15% in France and 30% in Germany. In low-calorie soft drinks, colas are the most popular, especially in the Northern European countries. For example, in Norway in 1990, 27% of carbonated sodas were 'light', which is almost the same percentage as 'light' colas consumed in the USA (Colas, 1990). The level of consumption of 'light' soft drinks is much lower in Southern Europe.

Table 8.1 Progress in soft drinks consumption in litres per capita (Millet, 1992)

Country	1976	1989
USA	108	176
Germany (FRG)	72	84
Belgium	60	72
The Netherlands	64	68
UK	34	71
Spain	49	65
Italy	24	44
France	26	34

The recent slowing down in growth of the low-calorie soft drinks market is partially due to the preference for the 'new age beverages' by young adults (Maxwell Jr., 1992). Such groups show preferences for what are called 'smart drinks', which are cocktails of soft drinks overdosed in vitamins, amino acids and oligo-elements. These 'smart drinks' are also consumed by older age groups hoping to limit the ageing effect. The benefits of these beverages may be doubtful (Maurice and La Fonta, 1992). In addition, sport drinks, caffeine-free formulations and soft drinks for diabetics should be taken into consideration in understanding the statistics and consumer preferences.

The importance of the consumption of non-alcoholic refreshing beverages in Europe and the USA are represented in Tables 8.2 and 8.3.

As already mentioned, the prospects for the soft drink market in general and the low-calorie sector in particular are moderate. However, despite the slow growth in the soft drink market, low-calorie soft drinks are gaining ground because of the innovation in formulation, packaging and processing.

8.2.2 Technical needs

It is difficult to replace sugar in soft drinks by artificial sweeteners without altering their quality of taste, flavour and ease of processing. In the formulation of low-calorie beverages, the balance between sweetness and sourness is critically important, from the taste profile point of view (McCormick, 1984). The 9 to 12% sugar concentration used in a normal soft drink requires less acidulant to reach the optimal balance than that needed for artificial sweeteners, especially when the taste profile is different from sucrose, as in the case of saccharin. Some formulations require the acidity to be adjusted by the use of a buffer, such as a salt of citric acid. Depending on the artificial sweetener used, the citric acid and citrate ratio may be changed (McCormick, 1984).

Table 8.2 Annual growth in the consumption of selected beverages in Europe (% annual growth) (Colas, 1990)

	1983–1988	1988–1989	Forecast 1989–1994
Carbonated beverages	+4.2	+5.9	+3.8
Juice drinks (+ powders)	+5.2	+9.5	+4.9
Fruit juices and nectars	−0.2	+6.8	+5.5
Concentrates (syrups)	−0.2	+2.4	+0.6
Bottled water	+6.4	+9.4	+4.6

Table 8.3 Annual growth (%) in consumption of selected beverages in USA (% annual growth) (adapted from Anon, 1992a)

	1983–88	1988–89	1989–90	1990–91	Forecast 1992–2000
Soft drinks	+6.0	+2.1	+2.6	+1.7	+2.0
Fruit beverages	+3.8	+4.3	+1.5	+6.6	+0.6
Bottled water	+17.5	+13.3	+9.5	+0.5	+6.2

The other noticeable difference resulting from the use of synthetic sweeteners in soft drinks is the reduced amounts of soluble solids as compared to sucrose, resulting in lower viscosity and altering the mouthfeel. In still beverages, such viscosity enhancers as food gums or modified starches are needed to stabilise the flavour, especially when low-density citrus oil is to be incorporated into a flavour emulsion to correct the palatability. An optimum sugar and artificial sweetener ratio is necessary in mixer drinks, such as tonic water or bitter lemon, which are mixed with spirits. An excess of sugar in such drinks could spoil the flavour.

The processing of soft drinks and powdered mixes poses specific problems. For example, the soft drinks require aseptic bottling and packaging for cold filling has to be previously sterilised by a combination of chemical (hydrogen peroxide) and heat treatments. The powdered mixes have to be packed in oxygen-free gas-tight containers (Anon, 1986). Ascorbic acid (vitamin C) as an antioxidant is often used. To improve the quality of soft drinks, membrane separation, reverse osmosis, ultrafiltration and microfiltration techniques are employed. The method of packaging of powdered drink mixes should be chosen to prevent caking due to absorption of moisture or by the presence of oxygen in the headspace of the package (McCormick, 1984). The most innovative sector in the soft drink industry in recent years was the growth in the use of plastic PET bottles, especially for diet carbonated beverages (Anon, 1986).

8.3 Formulation of low-calorie soft drinks

8.3.1 Sweetness

8.3.1.1 Formulation and optimal choice of the sweetener. Depending on the kind of low-calorie soft drink, and the objective of the formulation (zero-calorie, reduced-calorie and flavour), a single non-nutritive sweetener, a blend of sweeteners or of sugars and sweeteners can be used. Saccharin is rarely used alone because of its bitter aftertaste. This is not the case for aspartame which has an acceptable taste profile and can be used alone in carbonated drinks or mixed with saccharin. However, over a time period and at higher temperatures aspartame's stability decreases. Due to this factor, as well as cost considerations, it is generally used in combination with other synthetic or natural sweeteners.

Before the approval of aspartame in 1983, most low-calorie soft drinks used saccharin as the main sweetener. To mask the bitter aftertaste of saccharin, blends of saccharin and cyclamate or saccharin and sucrose were used (Wells, 1989). The US market used more than 70% of the saccharin and cyclamate mixture in low-calorie beverages. After 1983, it was found that small amounts of aspartame (7 mg l^{-1}) could be added to 330 mg l^{-1} of saccharin to produce an acceptable low-calorie soft drink. The taste requirements should not only be taken into account, but also the cost of formulation (Bakal and Nabors, 1986). Fructose and saccharin mixtures may be used to solve the taste problems but can be more expensive than other mixtures of sweeteners. However, it was recently discovered that fructose or high-fructose corn syrup (HFCS) improve the taste of soft drinks and permit substantial saving in artificial sweeteners (Kreuzberger, 1982).

The tendency after 1983 was to use increasing amounts of aspartame in soft drinks. The main reasons for its increased use were the quality of sweetness, the synergy with other sweeteners and the aggressive marketing of the company which imposed requirements to use a minimum quantity of aspartame (50%) in the blend, and to add the brand label on the package. Although the pH (3–3.5) of carbonated cola-type soft drinks is favourable for the sweetness stability of aspartame, the 'light' drinks, which comprise 51% of the low-calorie soft drinks market in France, use a mixture of the three major artificial sweeteners (aspartame, saccharin and acesulfame-K) (Millet, 1992). In the USA the same colas are sweetened with 100% aspartame. Emphasis should be given to the fact that 80% of world aspartame consumption occurs in the USA, with two thirds of the total employed in soft drinks. The use of aspartame can be understood for the American market in which the turnover of stocks is more rapid so that the decrease in sweetness intensity (due to its inherent instability) is not perceived.

The third most important artificial sweetener in the field of low-calorie soft drinks is acesulfame-K. The metallic aftertaste of acesulfame-K limits its use as a single sweetener. In addition, the acceptable daily intake (ADI) value of acesulfame-K is only 9 mg kg^{-1} bw. The heat stability of this synthetic sweetener allows its use, in preference to aspartame, to sweeten 'light' fruit beverages and nectars. The exclusive use of aspartame in the USA and the large preference of acesulfame-K in Germany is not only a matter of perceived product superiority but may be due to chauvinism, as the manufacturers of aspartame and acesulfame-K are, respectively American and German. An important characteristic of acesulfame-K is its synergism with other sweeteners. This product has been found to exhibit positive synergy when mixed with sucrose or aspartame (Von Rymon Lypinski, 1991). In addition to this synergism, acesulfame-K being considerably cheaper than aspartame, is used to reduce its cost.

8.3.1.2 Synergism.   The definition of 'positive synergy' is the perceived sweet taste of a mixture that is more intense than that of the individual constituents, at the same equi-sweet concentration as sucrose. The enhancement of sweetness is only observed when one or both components show an expansion behaviour (increase of intensity vs. concentration) (Bartoshuk, 1975). Interpretation of the sweetness of mixtures is influenced by the method of estimation of taste intensity. The 'pair comparison' method may mask the effect of synergy between stimuli which differ in more than one parameter, like the presence of an inherent bitterness in saccharin or acesulfame-K. The 'magnitude estimation' method when applied to mixtures showed that it is difficult to predict the sweetness from knowledge of the taste of its components (Larson-Powers and Pangborn, 1978). Moreover, this method is influenced by the quality of sweetness. Another procedure of estimation of synergy called the 'equimolar comparison' shows that the more active sweetener plays a dominant role (De Graaf and Frijters, 1987).

It was recently shown that the percentage of synergy of aspartame or acesulfame-K is high with fructose (30%), whereas sucrose shows about 13% maximum synergy with acesulfame-K and 12% suppression with aspartame (Mathlouthi and Portmann, 1993). The difference in synergy of these mixtures was attributed to the difference in compatibility of the hydration of the two components in the aqueous medium. The hydrophobic nature of aspartame and its influence on water structure is probably the origin of its negative synergistic effect. Acesulfame-K is probably more compatible with water structure and therefore exhibits positive synergy with other sweeteners (Mathlouthi and Portmann, 1993).

8.3.2   Bulking ingredients

Although the sweetness level of a low-calorie soft drink may be reached easily by use of artificial sweeteners, other properties of sugar like viscosity, specific gravity and humectancy are difficult to achieve using an artificial sweetener alone. The quality of taste of sucrose is due to many attributes rarely found in any one sweetener. These qualities are attributed to its concentration response function, viscosity, mouthfeel and flavour profile, which is derived from intensity time studies and the spatial selectivity in the mouth between the tongue and the oral cavity. It is almost impossible to obtain all these qualities without adding bulking agents like polyols, starch derivatives, gums, etc., to the formulation of low-calorie beverages. An overall descriptor of viscosity and texture is the degrees Brix (°Brix) of a beverage. A soft drink sweetened with sucrose has a 10.80 °Brix compared to 0.34 and 0.36 for aspartame and acesulfame-K, respectively, alone or in conjunction with maltol (Askar *et al.*, 1985). This means the reduction of specific gravity from 1.043 to 1.001 and the decrease of viscosity from 1.80 to 1.40 cP. Sucrose itself, or other sugars when mixed with saccharin, acesulfame-K or aspartame, give an improvement of the taste quality, contribute to correct the mouthfeel and other factors related to texture.

If the aim is to manufacture diet soft drinks, bulking ingredients other than sucrose should be used. There is a controversy regarding the energy value of low molecular weight polyols which have many of the properties required to replace sucrose, for example viscosity, mouthfeel and humectancy. Polyols are of interest as sweeteners because of their non-cariogenic and insulin independence properties. The nutritional and metabolic aspects of polyols such as sorbitol, mannitol and xylitol are discussed in chapter 3. They are generally credited with a lower nutritional value than sucrose. However, they have a laxative effect which limits their use in low-calorie soft drinks (Spada di Nauta and Camaggio Sancineti, 1991). Non-reducing disaccharides such as Palatinit, maltitol or lactitol, synthesised by the hydrogenation of their corresponding disaccharides, are of interest as low-calorie low-intensity sweeteners. They have a metabolisable energy of only 1.5 to 2.8 kcal g^{-1} which is almost half the energy of sucrose (Wurch and Anatharaman, 1989).

Polymeric carbohydrates like polydextrose, Lycasin® or inulin are suitable as dietary bulking agents. They are low-calorie, non-cariogenic and water soluble. Their increased viscosity allows the use of small amounts of these products to achieve the desired texture or mouthfeel for the diet beverage. They may also be used to stabilise flavours. About 3 to 5% (w/v) of polydextrose may be used in low-calorie soft drinks to give the mouthfeel and make the taste of an intense sweetener more rounded and less bitter (Murray, 1988). Polydextrose is only slightly degraded in the colon and its caloric value is estimated to be 1 kcal g^{-1}. It is well tolerated and it causes less gastrointestinal problems than low molecular weight polyols.

Lycasin® is a hydrogenated glucose syrup which is clear, colourless, sweet tasting (0.60× sucrose) and is composed of sorbitol (7%), hydrogenated oligosaccharides (60–70%) and polysaccharides (20%). These hydrogenated poly- or oligo-saccharides are less likely to be metabolised by microorganisms which makes them particularly suitable for low-calorie soft drinks. Their stability in solution is also increased by the absence of reducing groups. In addition, they are non-cariogenic, viscosity modifiers and have food preservative effect (Sicard and Leroy, 1983).

Oligofructoses and the polyfructose inulin are also of interest as bulking

Table 8.4 Relative characteristics and costs of commercial high-intensity sweeteners

Compounds	Sweetness (relative to sucrose)	Sweetness characteristics	Stability	Solubility in water	Synergism	Regulatory status	Relative cost (sucrose = 1)
Saccharin	300–600	Slow onset→ maximum→ persists	Generally stable in most food formulations	Na-salt readily soluble	Very good	Worldwide approval including USA (ADI 2.5 mg kg^{-1} bw)	0.02–0.03
Cyclamate	30–40	Slow onset→ lingering sweet–sour aftertaste	Good	Na-salt readily soluble	Very good	(ADI 11 mg kg^{-1} bw)	0.4–0.5
Aspartame	160–220 Average in soft drinks approx. 180×	Sugar-like taste	Stable in dry form. Most stable in solution at pH 4.3 Hydrolysis at pH 2–2.5	Only slightly soluble (1%, 25°C) Max. solubility at pH 2.2	Good	>18 countries (ADI 40 mg kg^{-1}bw)	0.9–1.2
Acesulfame-K	200×, 3% sucrose solution 100×, 6% sucrose solution	Bitter and synthesis aftertaste	Good	Good	Excellent	15 countries (ADI 9 mg kg^{-1} bw)	0.4–0.9
Sucralose	450×, 10% sucrose solution 650×, 5% sucrose solution	Sweetness time/intensity profile similar to sucrose	Good	Good	Good	Canada	0.5–0.9

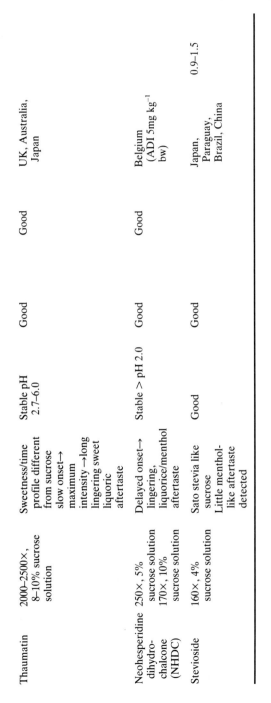

Thaumatin	2000–2500×, 8–10% sucrose solution	Sweetness/time profile different from sucrose slow onset→maximum intensity →long lingering sweet liquoric aftertaste	Stable pH 2.7–6.0	Good	Good	UK, Australia, Japan	
Neohesperidine dihydrochalcone (NHDC)	250×, 5% sucrose solution 170×, 10% sucrose solution	Delayed onset→ lingering, liquorice/menthol aftertaste	Stable > pH 2.0	Good	Good	Belgium (ADI 5mg kg^{-1} bw)	
Stevioside	160×, 4% sucrose solution	Sato stevia like sucrose Little menthol-like aftertaste detected	Good	Good	Good	Japan, Paraguay, Brazil, China	0.9–1.5

agents for use in soft drinks. The functional properties such as low and neutral sweetness, neutral colour and odour, and mouthfeel of inulin make it suitable for sugar substitution and intense sweetness adjustment in low-calorie soft drinks. The lack of reducing groups imparts heat stability. However, inulin may be hydrolysed at ambient temperature in beverages with a pH lower than 4.5, which limits its use in non-refrigerated soft drinks. The degree of hydrolysis remains lower than 10% in fruit beverages (pH 2.5–3.5), stored for three months at 5°C (Raffinerie Tirlemontoise, 1990).

8.4 Commercial artificial sweeteners

8.4.1 Introduction

The solution properties such as solubility, stability, taste quality and synergy are critically important for the application of an intense sweetener in a soft drink. In order to have a good acceptability in beverages a sugar substitute should have a sweetness profile similar to sucrose. The sweet taste should appear in a second or two and should remain for roughly 30 seconds. The delayed onset and the lingering of sweetness is undesirable in soft drink applications.

The sweetener must be chemically compatible with other ingredients of the beverage. It must also be stable under food processing conditions which would involve liquid phase, heating, fast freezing or freeze drying. For soft drinks the stability of the sweetener in a pH range from 2.5 to 8 is essential. Some of the properties of high-intensity sweeteners used commercially in low-calorie soft drinks formulations are discussed (Table 8.4).

8.4.2 Aspartame

Aspartame (α-L-aspartyl-L-phenylalanine-1-methyl ester) is 180–200 times sweeter than sucrose. Its solubility in water is about 1% at 25°C at pH 4.0. Its caloric value is 4 kcal g^{-1} and its acceptable daily intake (ADI) (WHO) is 40 mg kg^{-1} body weight (bw). The average aspartame content in a diet beverage is about 500 mg l^{-1} which is much less than the ADI of 2800 mg for an adult of 70 kg bw. The stability of aspartame in solution is affected by time, temperature and pH. For carbonated beverages, the pH range of 2.5–3.5 does not affect the sweetener to an appreciable degree. However, the combination of time and temperature is critical for the storage of beverages (Homler, 1984). The products of hydrolysis are aspartylphenylalanine and methanol, or in case of cyclisation, diketopiperazine, which is found at a maximum level of 4–5% in carbonated beverages, randomly selected (Vetsch, 1991). Short term pasteurisation and ultra high temperature (UHT) treatment of sweetened banana nectar was found to cause minor degradation for 20 seconds at 120°C (Djie *et al.*, 1991).

8.4.3   Acesulfame-K

Acesulfame-K is the potassium salt of 6-methyl-1,2,3-oxathiazin-4(3*H*)-one-2,2-dioxide. It has good solubility in water (270 g l^{-1} at 20°C). The relative sweetness is about 180–200 times that of sucrose at 3–4%. The value decreases rapidly to 100 at 6% sucrose solution (Von Rymon Lipinski, 1985). Acesulfame-K has no caloric value and its ADI is 0–9 mg kg^{-1} bw (WHO). As it has the same sweetness potency as aspartame, acesulfame-K may be used as a single sweetener in a beverage at a level of 500 mg l^{-1} which is close to the maximum 600 mg l^{-1} generally allowed in soft drinks. The thermal stability of acesulfame-K at pH above 3.0 is high, but when the pH is lower than 3.0 it is decreased, especially when the temperature is increased (Von Rymon Lipinski, 1985). Soft drinks sweetened with acesulfame-K may be pasteurised or sterilised without degradation of the sweetener.

8.4.4   Saccharin

Saccharin (2-sulphobenzoic-imide) or its sodium salt is the most common and oldest artificial sweetener. The sodium salt is readily soluble in water (1 g in 1.5 ml at 22°C). This solubility is increased in the presence of sugars or in an acidic medium (Fabiani, 1981). It is generally admitted that saccharin is 500 times sweeter than sucrose. The relative sweetness is affected by concentration, acidity and temperature. The sweet taste of saccharin is generally accompanied by a bitter aftertaste which may be masked by its use in combination with sugar or other sweeteners. Saccharin is known as a non-caloric, non-cariogenic, stable sweetener in soft drinks, even after thermal treatment by pasteurisation. However it is hydrolysed at low pH into 2-sulphobenzoic acid and 2-sulphamoylbenzoic acid. A loss of 20% saccharin in lemon juice stored at room temperature after 12 months has been observed, at 30°C it led to 16% hydrolysis in one month, and 34% after 6 months (Wells, 1989). The ADI limit of saccharin is 2.5 mg kg^{-1} bw which limits its use to approximately two cans of sweetened beverage per day.

8.4.5   Cyclamate

Salts of cyclohexylsulphamic acid are used in European countries but not in the USA as a sweetening agent for foods and beverages. Sodium cyclamate is soluble in water (20 g in 100 ml at 20°C). The sweetness potency is 30–40 times that of sucrose with an enhancement in acidic soft drinks. A sweet–sour lingering aftertaste may be detected at high concentrations. Its sweetness potency of 30 and ADI of 11 mg kg^{-1} bw (WHO) allow the use of only one can per day for an adult of 70 kg bw, which corresponds to 770 mg. Cyclamate is generally considered as a non-caloric, non-cariogenic sweetener. It can be used over a wide range of pH in soft drinks. Cyclamate is stable at normal and pasteurisation temperatures. However, the use of calcium cyclamate in the presence of fruit pectins or at high concentrations may cause gelling or precipitation problems.

8.4.6 Sucralose

4,1',6'-trideoxy-4,1',6'-trichloro-*galacto*sucrose (sucralose) is 650 times sweeter than sucrose (Hough and Khan, 1989). It is readily soluble in water (28% w/w, at 20°C), non-caloric, non-cariogenic, stable in acidic aqueous solutions such as soft drinks (Jenner, 1989). It is stable in most foods and beverages but it may be hydrolysed at low pH or degraded with elimination of hydrogen chloride in basic medium. The ADI is evaluated as 0–3.5 mg kg^{-1} bw (WHO). Sucralose has obtained approval in Canada and its approval is being sought in the USA and Europe.

8.4.7 Thaumatin

Thaumatin is an intensely sweet protein extracted from *Thaumatococcus danielli*, a West African plant. It is 2000–2500 times sweeter than sucrose (10%, w/w). It is commercialised by Tate and Lyle under the trade name Talin. It is very soluble in water (60%, w/w), its intensity–time sweetness profile is different from that of sucrose and it shows a lingering liquorice-like aftertaste. It has good stability in acidic aqueous solutions even after heating at 100°C, which is favourable for its utilisation in pasteurised soft drinks (Higginbotham, 1986). Its caloric value is 4 kcal g^{-1} but because of its high sweetness potency, its contribution to energy is negligible.

8.4.8 Neohesperidine dihydrochalcone (NHDC)

NHDC is a semi-synthetic non-nutritive sweetener derived from the biflavonoid neohesperidine present in grapefruit. Its solubility in water is about 0.40 to 0.50 g l^{-1} at 20°C. The relative sweetness of NHDC decreases from 250 to 170 for an equi-sweet sucrose solution, with concentration increasing 5 to 10% (Guadagni *et al.*, 1974). NHDC is stable in the range of pH and temperature generally used in the processing of soft drinks. NHDC is non-cariogenic and its caloric value is about 2 kcal g^{-1}. It is permitted in Belgium for the total replacement of sugar in lemonade (a maximum of 50 ppm). It has a pleasant taste and a lingering menthol aftertaste (Beerens, 1981).

8.5 Conclusion

The advent of aspartame, which provides a high quality sweetener, has dramatically transformed the consumer acceptability of low-calorie soft drinks. There is a real trend for 'healthier' food, and calorie reduction and health care in general has become a serious concern in the West. A synthetic sweetener can allow for some of this reduction without sacrificing palatability of food and beverages.

There are technical, health and commercial advantages in using mixed sweeteners. The availability of various sweeteners allows choice of a particular sweetener or a combination of sweeteners for a particular application. From a health point of view, daily intake of each will be lower if a combination of sweeteners is used. From a commercial point of view the cost could be reduced by mixing a high-quality, high-cost sweetener with a low-quality low-cost sweetener, provided the synergistic effect is favourable.

The potential of low-calorie, natural and synthetic sweeteners has been demonstrated but not yet fully realised. Investment in research and development could lead to better and 'healthier' foods and beverages.

References

Anon (1986) The success of soft drinks. *Food Manufacture*, **10**, 39–40, 92.
Anon (1992a) *Beverage World*, March 30.
Anon (1992b) Europe sees the life (the last word). *Food Engineering International*, 91.
Askar, A., Hassanien, F.R., Abd El-Fadeel, M.G. El-Saidy, S. and El-Zoghabi, M.S. (1985) Quality evaluation of two new non-nutritive sweeteners as substitutes for sucrose in jam and carbonated beverage. *Alimenta*, **24**, 27–37.
Bakal, A.I. and Nabors, L. O'B. (1986) Stevioside. In: *Alternative Sweeteners* (eds L. O'B. Nabors and R.C. Geraldi). Marcel Dekker, New York, Chapter 14, p. 295.
Bartoshuk, L.M. (1975) Taste mixtures: is mixture suppression related to compression?. *Physiol. Behav.*, **14**, 643–649.
Beerens, H. (1981) Sucres et édulcorants: Néohespéridine-dihydrochalcone et Aspartame. *Ann. Fals. Exp. Chim.*, **74**, 261–271.
Colas, C. (1990) Les soft, secteur de pointe. *Libre Service Actualités*, **26**, 36–39.
De Graaf, C. and Frijters, J.E.R. (1987) Sweetness intensity of binary sugar mixture lies between intensity of its components when each is tested alone and at the total molality of the mixture. *Chem. Senses*, **12**, 113–129.
Djie, Y.H., List, D. and Zache, U. (1991) Analysis of thermal degradation of aspartame during direct sterilisation/pasteurization of banana nectar. *Flüssiges Obst.*, **58**, 373–75.
Fabiani, P. (1981) Edulcorants de synthèse: Saccharine et dulcine. *Ann. Fals. Exp. Chim.*, **74**, 273–283.
Grimanelli, J.P. (1992) L'overdose de light. *Media*, **328**, 25–30.
Guadagni, D.G., Maier, V.P. and Turnbaugh, J.H. (1974) Factors affecting sensory thresholds and relative bitterness of limonin and naringin. *J. Sci. Food Agri.*, **25**, 1199–205.
Higginbotham, J.D. (1986) Talin protein (thaumatin). In: *Alternative Sweeteners* (eds L. O'B. Nabors and R.C. Geraldi). Marcel Dekker, New York, Chapter 6, p. 103.
Homler, B.T. (1984) Aspartame: Implications for the food scientist. *Food Technol.*, **38**, 50–55.

Hough, L. and Khan, R. (1989) Enhancement of the sweetness of sucrose by conversion into chloro-deoxy derivatives. In: *Progress in Sweeteners*, (ed. T.H. Grenby). Elsevier Applied Science, London, pp. 97–120.

Houghton, H.W. (1988) Low-calorie soft drinks 1988. In: *Low-calorie Products* (eds G.G. Birch and M.G. Lindley). Elsevier Applied Science, London, pp. 11–21.

Jenner, M.R. (1989) Sucralose: Unveiling its properties and applications. In: *Progress in Sweeteners* (ed. T.H. Grenby). Elsevier Applied Science, London, pp. 121–142.

Kreuzberger, H. (1982) Comparaison du coût de differents édulcorants dans la production des boissons non alcoolisées. *Bios*, **13**, 11, 3–5.

Larson-Powers, N. and Pangborn, R.M. (1978) Descriptive analysis of the sensory properties of beverages and gelatins containing sucrose or synthetic sweeteners. *J. Food Sci.*, **43**, 47–51.

Mathlouthi, M. and Portmann, M.O. (1993) Solution properties and the sweet taste of mixtures. In: *Synergy* (eds G.G. Birch, G. Campel-Platt and M.G. Lindley). Intercept, Andover.

Maurice, S. and La Fonta, M. (1992) La mode des smart-drinks, potion magique des raves. *Liberation*, 24 Août, 28–29.

Maxwell J.C. Jr., (1992) 1987–991 soft drink consumption trend. *Beverage Industry*, March, 2–15.

McCormick, R.D. (1984) Sweet/sour level is key to successful beverage formulations. *Prepared Foods*, June, 116–118.

Millet, P. (1992) Le light prend de la bouteille. *Revue de l'Industrie Agro-alimentaire*, **477**, 34–38.

Murray, P.R. (1988) Polydextrose. In: *Low Calorie Products* (eds G.G Birch and M.G. Lindley). Elsevier Applied Science, London, pp. 83–100.

Raffinerie Thirlemontoise (1990) *Oligofructoses*. Technical brochure.

Sfiligoj, E. (1992) The Beverage market index for 1992. *Beverage World*, May, 30–40.

Sicard, P.J. and Leroy, P. (1983) Mannitol, sorbitol and Lycasin, properties and food applications. In: *Developments in Sweeteners*, (eds T.H. Grenby, K.J. Parker and M.G. Lindley). Applied Science Publishers, London, Vol. 2, pp. 1–25.

Spada di Nauta, V. and Camaggio Sancineti, G. (1991) Los endulzantes caloricos como alternativa a la sacarosa: situacion actual y perspectivas. *Alimentaria*, Julio–Agosto, 67–77.

Vetsch, W. (1991) Aspartam functional propreties in food systems. *Sweet Taste Chemoreception Symposium*, Reims, September 1991.

Von Rymon Lipinski, G.W. (1985) The new-intense sweetener Acesulfame-K. *Food Chem.*, **16**, 259–269.

Von Rymon Lipinski, G.W. (1991) Sensory properties of acesulfame-K. In: *Acesulfame-K* (eds D.G. Mayer and F.H. Kemper). Marcel Dekker, New York, pp. 197–207.

Wells, A.G. (1989) The use of intense sweetners in soft drinks. In: *Progress in Sweeteners* (ed. T.H. Grenby). Elsevier Applied Science, London, pp. 169–214.

Wilkinson, S.L. (1988) Synthetic sweeten flavors market. *Chemicalweek*, November 23, 33–34.

Würch, P. and Anatharaman G. (1989) Aspects of the energy value assessment of the polyols. In: *Progress in Sweeteners* (ed T.H. Grenby). Elsevier Applied science, London, pp. 241–266.

Index

NEW BOOK INFORMATION

Low-Calorie Foods and Food Ingredients

Edited by **R Khan**, POLY-biós LBT, Trieste, Italy

This subject is amongst the hottest in food technology today. As people become more health conscious and willing to pay premium prices for the perceived benefit of low-calorie foods, the food industry has responded by devoting huge resources to the research and development of these products. This highly practical book provides an authoritative and comprehensive review of existing low-calorie food technology, and that which is near to providing products for the market.

Associated aspects also covered include safety, nutrition and physiology. The editor himself has patented an important sweetener, and he leads an international team of authors, all acknowledged experts in their individual fields.

This book is designed for: food industry research and development staff; technical and production managers;

Contents: Editorial introduction - *R Khan.* Low-calorie foods: relevance for body weight control - *J E Blundell and C de Graaf.* Regulatory aspects of low-calorie food - *G Urquhart and S V Molinary.* Low-calorie bulk sweeteners: nutrition and metabolism - *F R J Bornet.* Low-calorie bulking ingredients: nutrition and metabolism - *G Annison, C Bertocchi and R Khan.* Fat and calorie-modified bakery markets for fat-reduced foods - *M G Lindley.* Fat and calorie-modified bakery products - *R L Barndt and R N Antenucci.* High-intensity, low-calorie sweeteners - *L Hough.* Low-calorie soft drinks - *M Malthlouthi and C Bressan.* Index.

July 1993: 234x156: c.200pp:
48 line illus, 2 halftone illus:
Hardback: 0-7514-0004-1: £55.00

ORDER COUPON

Bulk Discount Hotline
071 522 9966

Send to: Direct Response Supervisor, Chapman & Hall Ltd, Cheriton House, North Way, Andover, Hants, SP10 5BE, England

UK orders: Tel: 0264 342923, Fax: 0264 364418

Overseas orders: Tel: UK +264 342830, Fax: UK +264 335973

If ordering in the USA, please contact: Ariel Hameon, Chapman & Hall Inc., 29 West 35th Street, New York, NY 10001, USA.

Tel: 212 244 3336, Fax: 212 563 2269

Also available from your bookseller.

Please send me:

☐ Copies of _____

☐ Copies of _____

Cheques with order/credit card orders will be sent carriage free within the UK. These orders can also be supplied, on request, within 24 hours for a charge of £8.50 per parcel within the UK. For all other orders add £3.50 per book for delivery in the UK or overseas surface mail and £9.50 for airmail. All published books are despatched within 3 days of receipt of order.

Refund policy: We will promptly refund payment for books returned within 30 days after receipt, provided they are in a saleable condition.

UK: Chapman & Hall, 2-6 Boundary Row, London, SE1 8HN, England.

Japan: Chapman & Hall Japan, Thomson Publishing Japan, Hirakawacho Nemoto Building, 6F, 1-7-11 Hirakawa-cho, Chiyoda-ku, Tokyo 102, Japan
FAX: 3 3 237 1459

Singapore: Thomson International Publishing, 38 Kim Tian Road, 01-05, Kim Tian Plaza, Singapore 0316.
FAX: 27 26 498

Australia: Chapman & Hall Australia, Thomas Nelson Australia, 102 Dodds Street, South Melbourne, Victoria 3205, Australia. FAX: 3 685 4199

India: R Seshadri, Chapman & Hall, 32 Second Main

made payable to Chapman & Hall

☐ Please invoice me/my company ☐ Please send me a **free catalogue** of publications
(Books will not be sent before we receive payment)

☐ Please charge £ _____ to my:

Visa \ Access \ Mastercard \ American Express \ Diners Club account

☐☐☐☐☐☐☐☐☐☐☐☐☐☐

Expiry Date _____ Signature _____

If name and address on your credit card differ from delivery address, please state

Name _____

Position/Dept _____

Organisation _____

Address _____

_____ Postcode _____

Tel: _____ Fax: _____

Date: _____ Signature: _____

Special Discount

Discounts are available on bulk orders (10 copies or more). Why not buy copies for your colleagues? Call our telephone hotline service on

071 522 9966

AJS special

05/93